D1597610

ANCIENT DISEASE
IN THE
MIDWEST

by

DAN MORSE

ILLINOIS STATE MUSEUM

Reports of Investigations, No. 15

Illinois State Museum

Springfield, Illinois

1978

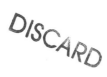

Published, 1969
Second Edition, Revised and Enlarged, 1978
ISSN 0360-0270
ISBN 0-89792-072-4

Printed by Authority of the State of Illinois
(P.O. 7388—2M—8-78)

CONTENTS

CONTENTS (Continued)

PLATES

FIGURES

TABLES

FOREWORD

Dr. Dan Morse, a physician by profession, is also a dedicated amateur archaeologist and a serious student of prehistoric physical anthropology. Beginning as a collector of artifacts, he has now become an ardent supporter of scientific archaeological research. It is not surprising that he, as a man of medicine, became intensely interested in the osteopathology of the skeletal material from the Dickson Mound excavation. He has studied these specimens and many others with great care and has consulted with paleopathologists and physical anthropologists as well as with colleagues in the medical field during his investigations.

Information gleaned from the study of ancient pathological skeletal remains not only extends the present knowledge of human bone disease but also increases the understanding of man's culture in prehistoric times. In this report Dr. Morse has discussed the abnormal bone changes brought about by disease, pointing out indicators and symptoms, as well as evidences of healing, and how to recognize them. Aware of the importance of good illustrations as adjuncts to the text, Dr. Morse personally financed the quality plates used in this publication. We are indebted to him for this contribution to the literature on prehistoric man—one more segment in the unending work of many to interpret life in prehistoric America.

Milton D. Thompson
Museum Director

April 1969

PREFACE

"Ancient Disease in the Midwest" could have been called just "Ancient Disease." The descriptions of the pathology apply to any location, but most of the examples in the illustrations are specimens recovered in the Midwest.

In the revised edition, two new chapters have been added: Chapter 10 on the X-ray; and Chapter 11, "Microscopic Analysis of Archaeological Bone," by Douglas Ubelaker. In addition, the Appendices now include a short review of osteology by Robert Dailey and Gina M. Comer and illustrated by Louis Tesar. It is hoped that this added material might increase the value of the book as a teaching aid in paleopathology.

January 1978   Dan Morse

ACKNOWLEDGMENTS

The author wishes to acknowledge the help received from the following individuals during the preparation of this manuscript:

The late Don Dickson, who had the forethought to collect and preserve the many pathological bone specimens which now have become the nucleus for the permanent collection of skeletal material of Dickson Mounds. His enthusiasm for the investigation of bone pathology can be likened to some of the diseases he studied, that is, it is "contagious" in that his interest spread to others.

Marion Dickson, who was always willing to give freely of his time and effort during the examination, recording and photographing of the many specimens; and Mrs. Don (Irene) Dickson for her cooperation and encouragement.

Dr. A. J. Novotny, Orthopedic Surgeon, Peoria, Illinois, who spent many hours with the author in reviewing and correcting the original draft.

Dr. Fred Decker, Chief of Radiology, Methodist Hospital, Peoria, and Dr. D. C. Dahlin, Department of Surgical Pathology, Mayo Clinic, Rochester, Minnesota, both of whom offered helpful suggestions.

Albert A. Dahlberg, D.D.S., Acting Director, Zoller Memorial Dental Clinic, and Research Associate of the Department of Anthropology, University of Chicago, who is the author of Chapter 8, *Dental Pathology*.

Dr. Georg Neumann, Department of Anthropology, Indiana University, who helped in many ways, furnished photographs and information, and made the skeletal collections of Indiana University available for examination; and King Hunter, Department of Anthropology, Indiana University, for his help and assistance in the examination of these specimens.

Others include: Dr. Charles Snow, Department of Anatomy, University of Kentucky Medical School; Alan Harn, Dickson Mounds, who supplied the artwork; Dr. Lent Johnson, Chief Orthopedic Pathologist, Armed Forces Institute of Pathology; Don Brothwell, British Museum of Natural History; Dr. J. Lawrence Angel and Dr. T. Dale Stewart of the Smithsonian Institution; Dr. Ivan Brown, Chief Pathologist, Methodist Hospital, Peoria; and Dr. Karl R. Sohlberg, Head Pathologist, Proctor Hospital, Peoria.

The author's appreciation goes to Milton Thompson, Director of the Illinois State Museum and members of his staff, under whose auspices this book is being published. Special thanks are due Miss Orvetta Robinson, Museum Librarian, and Dr. Paul Parmalee, Assistant Director.

Preliminary proofreading was done by Mrs. Josephine Long of the X-ray Department, Methodist Hospital, Peoria, and Mrs. Leonore Frank, Business Manager of the Peoria Tuberculosis Sanitarium, Peoria. Most of the typing was done by the author's wife, Ann Morse.

Assistance in archaeology was obtained from Dr. Joseph R. Caldwell, formerly Head Curator of Anthropology, Illinois State Museum, now Professor, Department of Anthropology, University of Georgia; Dr. Emily J. Blasingham, Head Curator of Anthropology, Illinois State Museum; Larry Conrad, formerly with the Illinois State Museum; and the author's son, Dr. Dan F. Morse, State Archaeological Survey, University of Arkansas.

Some of the material in Chapter 9 has appeared previously in *American Review of Respiratory Diseases* and in *Miscellaneous Papers in Paleopathology*, Museum of Northern Arizona. (See References Cited: Dan Morse, 1961, 1967.)

It is obvious that this book would never have been completed without the help of many. The author, however, accepts responsibility for all errors and realizes the probability of their existence. He further accepts sole responsibility for all opinions and conclusions and welcomes criticisms from the readers. These will be filed for future use in the event of reprinting.

ACKNOWLEDGMENTS FOR REVISED EDITION

In addition to the original acknowledgments, the author wishes to express his thanks to the following who contributed new material to this revised edition: Dr. Douglas Ubelaker, Associate Curator, Department of Anthropology, Smithsonian Institution, who is author of Chapter 11, "The Microscopic Analysis of Archaeological Bone"; Dr. Robert C. Dailey, Associate Professor, and Gina M. Comer, graduate student, Department of Anthropology, Florida State University, who composed Appendix 4 on osteology; Louis Tesar, Florida State Division of Archives, History and Records, who is responsible for most of the original illustrations in the section on osteology and in the chapter on the x-ray; and Margo Shand, professional illustrator, who provided other illustrations.

Recognition for their help in reviewing the chapter on x-ray goes to Wayne Haertling, Sales Representative, General Electric X-ray Company of Albany, Georgia, and to Mrs. Warren Whatley, Chief Technician, and to Dr. D. J. McCulloch, both of Radiology Associates, Tallahassee, Florida.

Others whose help is appreciated are Dr. Roy M. Hoover, retired orthopedic surgeon, Tallahassee, and Lou Causseaux, Department of Anthropology, Florida State University, for her typing and review of the entire manuscript.

Special thanks are due Dr. R. Bruce McMillan, Director of the Illinois State Museum, and to Miss Orvetta Robinson, Museum Librarian. Thanks are due also to Chad Braley and Don Merritt, Florida State University graduate students, and to John Goldsborough, National Park Service, for assistance in photography; and to Phillip Martin, Chairman of the Academic and Publication Board, Florida State University, for his overall advice.

INTRODUCTION AND DEDICATION

This book is dedicated to Don F. Dickson, who in 1927 originated the archaeological technique of excavating skeletal material whereby the burials are left in their original positions in the soil. Don, with his father, Thomas, and his uncle, Marion H., succeeded in uncovering and preserving for future exhibition over 200 burials. Dickson Mounds, first owned by the Dickson family, was purchased by the State of Illinois in 1945 and placed under the jurisdiction of the Department of Conservation. In 1965 the authority for its administration was transferred by legislative action to the Illinois State Museum under the Department of Registration and Education.

Though the efforts and genius of Don F. Dickson, Dickson Mounds has become internationally famous as a monument to the past. Don was interested in obtaining all information possible from these excavations, but his special interest was in physical anthropology and he made every effort to acquire knowledge concerning that too-often neglected portion of physical anthropology dealing with diseases and abnormalities. In the more than 35 years that he was associated with the Mounds, he succeeded in accumulating literally hundreds of pathological and abnormal specimens of skeletal remains. This vast storehouse of pathology is now the property of the State of Illinois and will be preserved for future study. Most of the illustrations in this book are of the pathological material collected by Don Dickson.

The Dickson pathological collection comes from all over the Midwest, but principally from two prehistoric Indian sites: (1) Dickson Mounds; and (2) Crable Cemetery, a Mississippian site located in southern Fulton County about 15 miles from Dickson Mounds. An archaeological summary of the Crable Site and Dickson Mounds is presented in the Appendix.

There are two reasons why a careful search for the pathological and the abnormal should always be a part of the study of excavated skeletons. The first and most obvious reason is that we should acquire *all* information about a culture. Disease plays an important role in shaping the lives of men and nations. In prehistoric times this role was at times major. The second reason is that the study of the thousands of available dried bone collections may increase our knowledge of *bone pathology*. It is essential that skeletal collections be well documented and all associations noted in order to place the material in its proper temporal and spatial aspect.

We close this introduction by quoting Don Dickson: "I would like you to take this thought home with you: You are not looking at a pile of skeletons; you are looking beyond them into the life of man. If you do this, you will also find a reason why people devote their lives to work such as this."

CHAPTER 1

GROSS PATHOLOGY OF DRIED BONE

In this report, the diagnosis of ancient disease is based almost entirely upon examination of dried skeletal remains. The clinician has at his disposal the history and the physical findings concerning a living patient, the course of the disease, plus many laboratory procedures for use in diagnosis. The anthropologist, confronted with only the bones, is at a distinct disadvantage. The x-ray is sometimes of help, and more investigative work is required before the usefulness of microscopic sections of dried bones can be evaluated.

Since most diseases have no detectable effect on the skeletal material, the anthropologist rarely can determine the cause of death. On the other hand, many minor bone changes, which can be tremendously significant, are not seen by the roentgenologist, the surgeon, or the pathologist. In addition, it is known that many of these minor bone changes will revert nearly to their original appearance with recovery from the disease or infection. If death occurs before reversion is accomplished, these minor bone changes assume great importance to the anthropologist.

The anthropologist with a knowledge of anatomy and medicine can become quite proficient in detecting pathology through experience in the examination of numerous specimens. He should not hesitate to seek the assistance of physician specialists, particularly the pathologist and the orthopedic surgeon. It is important to recognize what is antemortem and what abnormalities are caused by postmortem changes.

Postmortem Changes

Bone changes and damage occurring after death are not always easy to determine. Postmortem damage occurs for many reasons, the principal one being erosion and rotting due to the effects of the soil. The bone is much better preserved if the soil environment is neutral or slightly alkaline. Acidity of the soil severely damages the bone, frequently to such an extent that moving any piece of bone intact is almost impossible. The presence of moisture increases the chances of rotting. When the burial is close to the surface and the soil above it is porous, there is usually extensive softening of the skeletal material, making it extremely susceptible to breaking and chipping.

Much damage can occur also during the excavation, removal and transportation of the skeletal material to the laboratory. Special care and patience must be exercised in removing the skeleton, and one must be willing to spend a considerable amount of time in this endeavor. Other damaging elements are insects, roots and rodents.

Antemortem Bone Changes

Gross changes in the appearance of the bone caused by disease almost always incorporate two processes: destruction and regeneration. The healing process or regeneration of live bone varies greatly according to the causative agent. For example, in pyogenic osteomyelitis the regeneration of bone is tremendous; in tuberculous osteitis regeneration is very minimal; and in some tumors, as in multiple myeloma, the regeneration is practically zero. If there is no evidence of regeneration, then it must be assumed that changes in practically every instance are postmortem.

Bone resorption is a part of healing in either disease or trauma. Formation of new bone plus resorption of old bone is the method by which osseous tissue reshapes and remolds itself in an attempt to gain a functional recovery. In reaction to disease or injury, bone resorption proceeds at a faster rate than repair; consequently, a disease of moderately brief duration may show only resorption and no evidence of regeneration. Furthermore, early repair is very poorly calcified. This condition can be seen on the x-ray of living patients but might not be evident in archaeological material.

If the individual lives after an injury, the body will form new bone in an effort to repair the damage. If the injury caused immediate death, there would be no signs of healing. In this case, one must take into consideration the appearance and location of the bone wound.

Bone Regeneration

The gross appearance of regenerating bone varies considerably. One of the most common appearances is the occurrence of many tiny pits of destruction, with the edges showing tiny nodules of new regenerating bone. Sometimes there are areas of large, irregularly shaped, destructive cavities surrounded by variously sized bony spicules and nodules. If destruction completely isolates a portion of bone, cutting it off from its blood supply, that portion will die. This portion, called a sequestrum, may be very small or it may include the entire shaft of a long bone.

In response to an irritation, usually caused by severe soft-tissue infections, layers of new bone will be deposited on the surface. The new surface thus formed can be smooth or irregular. When the new bone deposits (which can be identified as localized thickening, usually with sharply demarcated boundaries) show an irregularly roughened surface, sometimes with cavities of various sizes, the process is still active at the time of death. If the new bone surface is smooth and the edges of any depression and nodules present are rounded, the process can be considered healing or healed.

At times the bone responds to an irritating infection by a great increase in its density. This increased density, called hyperostosis, can cause a part of the bone to become enlarged and much heavier. It will occur in certain forms of chronic osteomyelitis and also as a response to trauma.

The effects of pressure in stimulating bone to react is seen in some cases of scoliosis. The cancellous bone in those portions of the vertebral bodies which bear most of the support will thicken and become more dense. Occasionally an entire bone will become enlarged as a response to increased pressure and stress. An example of this would be pronounced hypertrophy of a fibula in order to take over the weight-bearing function of the tibia, lost because of an ununited fracture.

In healing fractures, the bone will not only regenerate in an attempt to unite but will subsequently go through a reshaping and remolding process to compensate for the stresses of use. This same remolding (formation of new bone and resorption of old bone) is an important factor in attempted healing of bone destruction caused by disease.

Osteophytes, trabeculations, and nodules occurring on joint edges and surfaces are a part of aging and, if minor, are of very little significance when occurring in older individuals. Localized areas of tiny to moderately sized pitting, or shallow ulcer-like depressions surrounded by nodular and/or trabecular regeneration is a common finding especially in younger individuals. This condition has been described in man and monkeys and is given the name *criba orbitalia* because of its frequent occurrence in the orbits; but the same condition will occur in other parts of the skeleton (Plate 23,F). The cause is unknown but thought by many to be due to a nutritional deficiency.

Changes in Bone Density

Bone contains two substances: *osteoid tissue*, produced by bone cells called osteoblasts, which forms the bone matrix and acts as a framework, and the *mineral content*, consisting of calcium and phosphorus, which gives the bone strength and rigidity.

Osteoporosis, a decrease in the density of the bone because of a decrease in the matrix, can occur when there is a decreased production of bone matrix by the osteoblasts or an increased resorption of the matrix by another type of bone cell called the osteoclasts. In osteoporotic bone the individual trabeculi in the matrix have decreased in volume and in number and therefore contain less calcium and phosphorus because of the decrease in the total bone mass. With the bone now more porous, much lighter, and more brittle, the possibility of fracture is increased. There are many causes of osteoporosis: disuse, old age, malnutrition (protein deficiency), postmenopause, endocrine disturbances, anemias, and many chronic and debilitating diseases which severely restrict the individual's activity. Prolonged disuse of any portion of the body results in the development of osteoporosis. This occurs when a limb is immobilized because of an injury or disease. The process is reversible if activity is resumed. Old age is probably the most frequent cause of osteoporosis. As one gets older, bone structure will thin; but there is no measurable proportionate relationship of age to the degree of osteoporosis present. It is believed that a decrease in hormone secretions is the real cause of osteoporosis in the aged, along with disuse and improper diet.

Osteomalacia differs somewhat from osteoporosis. The mineral content of the bone is very much less than normal for the amount of matrix. The most common cause of osteomalacia is vitamin D deficiency, as in rickets. The predominating sign is a lack of rigidity of the bone so that it will bend easily, resulting in fractures and severe deformities. In severe cases where the mineral content is radically deficient, the bone is flexible and can be bent like hard rubber. This extreme condition probably never will be encountered in archaeological material.

Osteopetrosis, an excessive density of the bone (generalized), is a rare hereditary condition in which the medullary cavities are filled with calcified cartilage (see Chapter 6).

Osteosclerosis, localized areas of increased density, is characterized by an increase in the volume of the bone and its mineral content. It occurs in many conditions ranging from infections to trauma. Some specific infections, such as syphilis, can stimulate the bone to thicken and become more dense. Overlying soft-tissue infections can have a similar effect.

CHAPTER 2

CLASSIFICATION OF ANCIENT DISEASE

Obviously, the pathology and abnormalities existing in prehistoric bone are of the greatest value when the origin of the specimen is known and documented. If pathology can be identified as to the time and culture, then one can get some idea of *incidence* by comparison with previously reported cases and with cases that will be discovered in the future.

An estimation of the degree of disability of the individual who had a disease or abnormality is important. How a disabled individual adjusted to his environment, how his associates tolerated his sickness, and whether the community offered any aid, such as splinting or surgery, to a badly injured person are questions difficult to answer; but the mere presence of identifiable chronic disease which must have persisted for a long time indicates some sort of adjustment and tolerance. There have been instances where certain types of artifacts are found in the male grave and different types of artifacts in the female grave. In the Emmons Cemetery the grave of a severely deformed male hunchback contained pottery bowls which elsewhere in the same cemetery were almost entirely limited to female burials (Morse, Morse, and Emmons 1961). (See Plate 29,F.) In another part of the Emmons Site, an elderly man with a fractured leg and spondololysis was buried with the skeleton of a young child, suggesting that he may have had the responsibility of caring for the infant in order to carry his share of labor (Plate 3,A).

Mass burials, encountered in certain sections of central Illinois, suggest epidemics or warfare although the cause of death was not determined by examination of the bones. Group burials in the same grave are encountered frequently. At Dickson Mounds there are several, probably indicating either an epidemic or human sacrifice. The relationship of the individuals to one another in these group burials makes it quite certain that all were buried at the same time.

It cannot be emphasized too strongly that an examination of the entire skeleton is always necessary. Depositories or registries for bone pathology should insist on having all available skeletal material from each specimen, even though grossly there is only localized disease. This is important for two reasons: one is that an x-ray examination and microscopic sectioning may show abnormalities not seen by the eye alone, and the second is that undoubtedly new techniques will be developed in the future, such as chemical analysis and special bone precipitation tests. If possible, those looking for evidence of pathology should examine the skeleton *in situ,* for much can happen during excavation and transportation to the laboratory.

Since many different diseases can produce identical structural changes in bone, it is rarely possible to determine the specific cause when attempting to diagnose skeletal material; therefore, any classification of pathology based solely on cause will not be completely satisfactory. Some disease conditions do affect the bone in a specific manner, especially if one takes into consideration the localized appearance and the distribution throughout the skeleton. In addition, frequency of occurrence of similar lesions in any one excavation area can be helpful.

It is not intended that this book be all-inclusive. Liberal use of literature on bone diseases is indicated. The following classification appears to be best for our purpose:

TRAUMA
ARTHRITIS
INFLAMMATION OF BONE
TUMORS
ANOMALIES
DENTAL PATHOLOGY
SPECIFIC DISEASES

CHAPTER 3

TRAUMA

Traumatic lesions are perhaps the most common abnormal conditions seen in prehistoric bones. Results of trauma can be classified as: (1) fractures, (2) crushing injuries, (3) bone wounds caused by sharp instruments, (4) osteosclerosis which can occur with or without fractures, (5) dislocations, and (6) surgery.

Fractures

Fractures of the bone are caused by trauma. They can be classified as closed, open, complete, incomplete, comminuted, and pathological—or a combination of these. A *closed*, or simple, fracture is one in which the skin has not been broken and there is no connection between the point of fracture and the outside of the body. An *open*, or compound, fracture is one in which there is such a connection, caused either by a penetrating foreign body breaking the skin or by a fracture-end piercing the skin from the inside. A *complete* fracture is one in which the ends of the bone are separated; in an *incomplete* fracture the break does not go entirely through the bone. This sometimes happens in young children and is called a "green-stick" fracture. In a *comminuted* fracture there are multiple breaks or splintering so that one or more fragments become detached from the main bone. A *pathological* fracture is a break in a bone which has been weakened by some type of bone disease—such as cysts, tumors, osteomyelitis, etc. Fractures can occur with or without infection. It is rare for a closed fracture to become infected; therefore, when infection is in evidence in a dried bone specimen, the implication is that it was an open or compound condition.

Broken bones can further be classified as union or non-union. The causes of non-union are principally inadequate immobilization, wide separation of bone ends, and infection. Occasionally the bones will be united not by bone tissue but by a fibrous tissue, resulting in the formation of what is called a false joint or pseudoarthrosis. In pseudoarthrosis, the two ends of the bone may become quite smooth so that they articulate with each other, and often a cartilage plate and synovial membrane will form. In union, the healing can be satisfactory, resulting in a good functional bone, or unsatisfactory, resulting in disability. Unsatisfactory healing includes such things as:

(1) Shortening or over-riding, where the fractured bone becomes shorter than the opposite side.

(2) Angular deformity, where there is a sharp angle or bend in the bone at its healing point.

(3) Rotation deformity, with one end of the broken bone twisting either to the right or left.

The mechanism by which a fracture heals is as follows: During the trauma blood vessels are ruptured and a blood clot or hematoma occurs in the vicinity of the break. In the past it was thought that a callus was formed within the clot, which first consisted of cartilage and later bone. Recent opinion, however, is that the callus will form on adjacent tissues and a clot is not only unnecessary but actually can be the cause of unsatisfactory union or non-union (Collins 1966). The callus is usually large at first, and an excessive amount of bone may be produced. After the fragments are united, resorption takes place and the callus becomes smaller. Frequently a combination of resorption and production of new bone occurs simultaneously so that the bone becomes reshaped; and sometimes it is quite difficult to tell that there has ever been a fracture. This reconstructive process will occur even in badly aligned fractures and may continue for months or even years after the injury. In young people, reshaping in severe over-riding fractures can include actual lengthening of the entire bone so that there may be no significant shortening. This lengthening is brought about by the

TABLE 1

PREHISTORIC FRACTURES

SITE LOCATION CULTURE	NO. OF INDIVID- UALS	NO. OF FRAC- TURES	BURIAL NUMBER	LOCATION OF FRACTURE	UNION	DEFORMITY	DISABILITY
Steuben Illinois Late Hopewell	54	3	16 37 ”	R. Humerus Thoracic (12) Lumbar (1)	Yes Yes Yes	Slight angle None None	None None None
Emmons Illinois Mississippian	83	2	29 12	R. Femur R. Zygoma	Yes Yes	None None	None None
Robinson Tennessee Late Archaic	51	5	5 ” 24 ” 30	R. Femur R. Tibia L. Ulna L. Radius L. Humerus	Yes Yes Yes Yes Yes	2 in. short — None None Slight angle	Limp — None None None
Dickson Mounds Illinois Mississippian (in situ)	248	7*	25 7 106 ” 212 58 21	R. Humerus 2nd Rib R. R. Clavicle Skull (frontal) R. Humerus R. Ulna R. Tibia	Yes Yes Yes No Yes Yes Yes	None None None Healing at time of death None None Slight angle	None None None Healed infection None
Dickson Mounds Illinois Mississippian 1966 Excavation	83+	4	267 254 243 ”	Lumbar (2) R. Fibula L. 9th Rib L. 10th Rib	Yes Yes Yes Yes	None None None None	None None None None
Klunk Illinois Hopewell with some Archaic and Late Wood- land (Bluff)	395	20	C30-20 ” C30-52 C30-58 C31-15 C35-16 C35-23 ” C36-59 ” C36-64 C36-5 ” ” ” C37-20 C40-95 C40-64 ” C40-103	L. Tibia L. Fibula L. 11th Rib R. 3rd Metatarsal R. Humerus Skull depressed (frontal) R. 2nd Metacarpal R. 3rd Metacarpal R. Ulna L. Ulna L. Clavicle L. 8th Rib L. 9th Rib L. 10th Rib L. 11th Rib Head of R. Radius R. Nasal Bone R. Rib L. Rib R. Rib	Yes Yes Yes Yes Yes Yes Yes Yes Yes Yes Yes Yes Yes Yes Yes Yes No Yes Yes Yes	None None None None None None None None None None Overriding None None None None Traumatic Arthritis Healing at time of death None None None	None None None None None Healed None None None None None None None None None None None None

*Not true incidence because many skeletons are not completely excavated.   (Continued on next page)

TABLE 1 (concluded)

SITE LOCATION CULTURE	NO. OF INDIVID- UALS	NO. OF FRAC- TURES	BURIAL NUMBER	LOCATION OF FRACTURE	UNION	DEFORMITY	DISABILITY
Morse Illinois Late Archaic	62+	7	772-1	R. Radius	Yes	None	None
			"	L. Ulna	Yes	None	None
			772-7	R. Femur	Yes	½ in. short	None
			772-10	R. Femur	Yes	None	None
			772-29	Skull (frontal)	Yes	None	None
			Mound fill	L. Ulna	Yes	None	None
			707-16	Skull depressed (frontal)	Yes	Well healed	—
Vandeventer Illinois Mississippian	?	6	Van	R. Maxilla	Yes	Well healed	None
			"	R. Ulna	No	False joint	None
			"	R. Femur	Yes	Slight overriding	None
			"	R. Fibula	Yes	None	None
			"	R. Tibia	Yes	Slight overriding	None
			"	L. Clavicle	Yes	Slight shortening	None
Ogden Illinois Hopewell	?	4	HC3	R. Humerus	Yes	Osteosclerosis	None
			J13	R. Tibia	Yes	None	None
			IJ12	R. Tibia	Yes	None	None
			82	R. Tibia	Yes	Slight angle	None
Crables Illinois Mississippian (Dickson Mounds Collection)	?	13	K1	R. Fibula	Yes	None	None
			—	R. Fibula	Yes	None	None
			—	R. Radius	Yes	Overriding	Arm 1 in. shorter
			—	5th L. Rib	Yes	None	None
			—	6th L. Rib	Yes	None	None
			—	7th L. Rib	Yes	None	None
			K1085	R. Humerus	Yes	Slight angle	Arm ½ in. shorter
			K1219	L. Femur	Yes	Slight angle	None
			K648	R. Femur	Yes	Healed infection	None
			K1580	R. Tibia	Yes	None	None
			K12198	R. Fibula	Yes	None	None
			K1656	L. Tibia	Yes	None	None
			K1665	R. Tibia	Yes	Osteosclerosis	None
Dickson Illinois Mississippian (pre-excavation)	?	7	168	L. Fibula	Yes	None	None
			B-4	L. Tibia	Yes	None	None
			80	L. Femur	Yes	Slight angle and bowing	None
			D518	L. Humerus	Yes	None	None
			167	R. Humerus	Yes	Angle and Osteosclerosis	None
			87	Neck of Femur	Yes	Angulation	Limp
			—	L. Radius	Yes	None	None

growth of the bone at its epiphyseal ends. In adult life after closure of the epiphysis, lengthening in this manner is presumed impossible; but the number of over-riding fractures found in prehistoric material where the two long bones are approximately the same length suggests that even the adult fractured bone might be able to lengthen itself. There is some evidence that this may take place through a stimulation of the cartilage plates at the ends of a fractured long bone so as to produce new bone and new length (Johnson 1959, and Garn et al 1967). The present thinking is that the amount of new length is very minimal and therefore of little assistance in correcting a shortening deformity. In addition, it is possible to conceive that bony bridging between fracture ends may itself produce some additional lengthening.

Of the many fractures viewed by the author among prehistoric skeletal material of the Midwest, the vast majority showed union with good functional results. Only six out of 76 (7.9%) showed any disability of significance after healing. (See Table 1.) This certainly leaves one with an impression of the unusual ability of injured bone to heal itself. Whether the midwestern prehistoric Indians used splints or some other method to create immobility is a question that we cannot answer. It is very likely that early ambulation must have been the rule and quite certain that such things as pinning, open surgery, and possibly traction were nonexistent. Many reports in early literature demonstrate beyond a doubt that historic Indians had knowledge of how to treat fractures (Densmore 1926-27; Hrdlicka 1908; Mooney and Olbrechts 1932; Stevenson 1901-02; Stone 1962). These reports contain descriptions of certain individuals in some tribes who became quite skilled in setting fractures, using splints, and even reducing dislocations. It is safe to assume that their ancestors were capable of performing the same skills.

Crushing Injuries

Crushing injuries can be caused by falls or by blows from large and heavy objects and blunt weapons. Most skull fractures probably could be classified as crushing injuries. Other common sites of crushing injuries are the hands and feet. If the blood supply is severely limited by the injury, then healing may be delayed. A large callus sometimes forms in order to obtain a union, often resulting in a considerable amount of bone regeneration, fusion and deformity. In fractures of the skull infection is rather common because the same injury that caused the fracture may also break the skin and thus introduce infectious organisms. If a defect in the bone occurs in the skull as a result of the fracture, with or without infection, usually an open space or hole remains for the remainder of the individual's life even though the bone becomes completely healed. It appears that the surrounding bone is unable to regenerate and fill the hole or gap. At times healed depressed fractures will result in the formation of a cup-like depression on the surface of the bone.

Determining the age of a fracture in a dried bone specimen is difficult. If death occurs immediately, then the edges of the broken bone will be sharp with no evidence of healing, callus formation, smoothing or bone regeneration. In about ten days after injury, depending on the location of the break and age of the individual, an x-ray of a living patient and/or the direct visualization by a surgeon may show the bone ends of a fracture to be smooth and rounded—and in two to three weeks some evidence of callus formation may appear. In the case of infection, bone destruction may become apparent in an x-ray in about the same length of time. In documented amputation and postmortem specimens of dried bones described with photographs in a series of books called *The Surgical History of the War of the Rebellion* by Otis and Huntington there is no apparent evidence of bone healing or, in cases of infection, of bone destruction within a month to six weeks after injury. It is evident that the early changes seen in x-rays may be lost in the dried specimens. Final healing of a fracture or a bone infection can take many months or years.

Bone Wounds Caused by Sharp Instruments

The best evidence that a wound was caused by a sharp instrument is the presence of the instrument still imbedded in the bone. If the adjacent bone shows any signs of healing, then it can be assumed that more than a few weeks passed between the injury and death.

Longitudinal grooves or scratches in the bone indicate contact with sharp weapons, providing postmortem changes can be ruled out.

Occasionally an elliptically-shaped hole is found in a flat or long bone which may have been caused by penetration of a knife or spear point. According to Wilson (1901), who wrote about arrow wounds in *Early Indian Encounters*, an arrow can enter a bone at a great velocity and either become imbedded in the bone or pass completely through it, leaving no evidence of splintering at either the point of entrance or exit.

Whether scalping occurred among prehistoric Indians has not been determined. According to Mooney in *Handbook of American Indians* (1910), scalps were taken by the historic Indians as trophies, usually from dead enemies, and an increase of the scalping practice over a great part of central and western United States was a direct result of the encouragement through scalp bounties offered by colonial and other governments. There have been reports of several examples of skull wounds supposedly the result of scalping in prehistoric times. These are not too convincing, for it appears from early descriptions that it would be unusual and unnecessary for the skull to be damaged during a scalping. If skull damage was present, it would be difficult to distinguish whether the victim had been scalped or had received an abundance of nonspecific knife wounds. Snow (1941) reports a skull found at Moundsville in Alabama (Middle Mississippian) with a groove of osteitis completely encircling the top of the cranial vault. If this was scalping, it was an unsuccessful attempt; for if the scalp had been removed and the Indian lived, then the osteitis would cover the entire area which had been denuded. Neumann (1940) reports a case of "scalping" from the Crable Site in Illinois (Mississippian). Evidence of scalping in this case was attributed to the presence of many longitudinal cuts in the frontal and occipital areas of the skull (Plate 7,C). Neumann states that death had probably been caused by four celt blows which fractured the parietals and crushed the right side of the skull.

Osteosclerosis

Hypertrophy and increase in density of the bone are a common occurrence not only in infection but also in trauma. In many fractures, especially in those with considerable deformity, osteosclerosis is found not only close to the point of fracture but sometimes involving the entire bone. In angular deformity, osteosclerosis is more prominent on the concave side, as if to give additional strength to the side that has the more strain. In some prehistoric skeletons only a single bone shows marked osteosclerosis. The reason for this is not known but in the absence of any evidence of previous fractures, it is assumed to be a response to some sort of trauma (see Plate 10,C,D,E).

Dislocations

Dislocation in the prehistoric Indian was undoubtedly a common occurrence. Diagnostic bone changes would be uncommon except in those nonreduced cases. It is inconceivable, however, that the Indian did not learn how to reduce most dislocations. Pulling the finger, straightening the elbow, or manipulating a shoulder could correct the injury. One could expect severe dislocations to occur less frequently in prehistoric times, because of the absence of modern apparatus such as trains, airplanes, automobiles and tractors, which are capable of producing a terrific amount of force. It takes an unusual amount of force to produce many dislocations, especially those of the hip, knee, wrist and ankle.

Dislocations occur most frequently in young adults and the middle-aged. In the very young, a violent force is more likely to cause an epiphyseal slipping or separation. In the elderly, the same type of force would result in a fracture.

Dislocations of the fingers or toes can usually be easily reduced by a tug or they will reduce themselves. Dislocation of vertebrae are almost always incompatible with life because of cord injury. Dislocation of the hip can be congenital or traumatic. Congenital dislocations are characterized by a narrowing of the acetabulum. A bilateral congenital case, in a Late Archaic burial, is illustrated in Plate 6,B. An unreduced traumatic hip dislocation can result in atrophy of the leg bones, a deformity of the head of the femur, narrowing of the acetabulum, or a hollow depression on the surface of the ilium to accommodate the displaced head of the femur as shown in Plate 6,A.

Dislocation of the shoulder is the most common of all dislocations but not too difficult to reduce. If a chronic persistent dislocation did occur, then many bone changes will be evident such as atrophy, osteoporosis, a filling-in of the glenoid fossa, and in some cases a hollow depression where the displaced head of the humerus rests on a portion of the scapula.

Surgery

Many accounts in early literature testify to the fact that historic Indians had a knowledge of surgery. Setting bones, applying splints, reducing dislocations, bloodletting, tooth extraction by blows from blunt weapons or pulling with a sinew, applying heat to dental cavities, draining abscesses, removing arrow points,* and even amputations were practiced by historic Indians. There is no reason to believe that their ancestors were not capable of the same skills.

Scarifiers have been found in village sites and graves of prehistoric Indians, suggesting that these instruments (consisting of a number of bone slivers with sharp ends) could have been used for bloodletting (Plate 10,A).

A case of possible amputation (Plate 6,C,D) was found at the Klunk Site by Gregory Perino, working for the Gilcrease Foundation. The case was a 40-year-old male (Archaic Culture) with a missing right hand. The end of the right radius is enlarged to form a ball-like formation of bone. This would presume amputation, but disarticulation caused by trauma cannot be ruled out (see also Plate 21,B,C).

Two cases of possible jaw surgery are pictured (Plates 4,1 and 27,B). One is from the Vandeventer Mississippian Site in Brown County, Illinois, and the other is a Late Wood-

land burial (Indian Mound Park) in Adams County, Illinois. In defense that these two jaw cases could have involved surgery, C. M. Stevenson (1901-1902) described a Zuni Indian who had a healed fistulous opening in his cheek resulting from the surgical removal of a fragment of bone following a fracture of the left maxilla.

The antiquity of trephining, which is making a hole in the skull using surgical instruments, has been firmly established both in the Old and the New World. The vast majority of instances of trephining discovered in the New World have been from Peru, where hundreds of cases have been reported. In 1958, in an article on Stone Age skull surgery by Dr. T. D. Stewart, the author suggested that there are in existence over 1,000 Peruvian trephined skulls, stating that he himself had personally examined over two hundred.

Prehistoric trephining in the Midwest has not been proven. There have been some cases that the excavators have termed trephination; but desire on the part of the discoverer may overshadow the logic that a hole in the skull will more often be caused by trauma or infection than by surgery. If skull surgery were the custom in any one culture, one would expect to find many examples; but such is not the case in midwestern skeletal collections.

Whenever a skull defect due to injury or disease occurs in such a manner that a fragment of bone is completely isolated, the surrounding cranial bone can not regenerate to fill the defect. Furthermore, when healing occurs, the hole can actually become larger.

Although it is impossible to ascertain in all instances that a hole is caused by surgery or trauma, certain characteristics in the appearance of a cranial wound would indicate that trephination was the most probable cause. These are listed as follows:

(1) Crosshatched cuts surrounding the opening (Plate 9,A).
(2) Multiple holes in various stages of healing (Plate 9,B).
(3) A rectangular or square-shaped skull defect, suggesting that such a pattern would unlikely result from a traumatic fracture (Plate 9,C). A nearly perfect circle would slightly favor surgery as its cause.

---

*In 1883, a Dr. W. Thorton Parker described an Indian method of removing arrowpoints when imbedded in the wound. He states that a willow stick is split, the pith scraped out and the ends rounded so they may readily follow the arrow track. The stick is then introduced so as to reach and cover the barbs. It is then adjusted and bound to the arrowshaft, and all are withdrawn together (Wilson 1901).

(4) An area of bone osteitis surrounding the opening with straight borders forming an angular pattern, suggesting that the scalp flaps were removed or turned back by the surgeon in order to gain bone exposure. Dr. Frederick E. Jackson (1966) made the following statement: "The importance of soft-tissue coverings in the prevention of infection is emphasized by the fact that denudation of the skull is often followed by ischemic necrosis, osteitis and sequestration of bone." (Plate 9,D).

(5) Evidence that the operation was accomplished by the drilling of multiple holes around the section of bone which was removed (Plate 9,E).

Pedro Weiss (1958) states that there were three principal techniques used by prehistoric Peruvian surgeons: cutting, scraping and drilling. He shows a photograph of one skull where all three techniques were used.

CHAPTER 4

ARTHRITIS

Arthritis is a disease abnormality involving one or more joints. Many different classifications of arthritis and rheumatism have been proposed by authors and organizations. None of these appear to be satisfactory—especially for archaeological specimens. Most of them depend a great deal on etiology and clinical findings and, in an effort to be all-inclusive, are lengthy and complicated. For example, the classification tentatively accepted by the American Rheumatism Association contains 13 main headings and some 94 subheadings.

The classification of arthritis presented here is oversimplified and contains many omissions. However, in the examination of dried bone alone, certain pathological changes may be observed which would indicate that the disease entity could fall into one of the following categories:

(1) Degenerative joint disease
  (osteoarthritis)
(2) Vertebral osteophytosis
(3) Traumatic
(4) Rheumatoid
(5) Ankylosing spondylitis
(6) Infectious

There are two types of joints. *Synarthrosis* is a union of bones by some substance such as fibrous tissue, cartilage, or even bone itself. There is little or no movement and no true joint space. Examples are sutures of the skull and the symphysis pubis. *Diarthrosis* consists of two or more bone ends or joint surfaces covered with an articular cartilage and the entire joint is enclosed in a fibrous articular capsule, the inner surface of which is covered by a synovial membrane (Fig. 1). Examples are knee, elbow, hip, shoulder, temporomandibular, and the articulations between the articular processes of the vertebrae.

Degenerative Joint Disease

Evidence of degenerative joint disease or osteoarthritis is encountered very frequently in skeletal collections. It is considered a sign of aging, and nearly everyone will acquire it if he lives long enough. Although efforts have been made to use the degree of osteoarthritis as a measure of age, any such estimation would be only approximate and quite unreliable due to the great variation in individuals as to the time of development and the extent of degenerative joint disease.

The initial pathological changes occur in the articular cartilage. Degeneration of the cartilage results in a thinning and erosion. The bone beneath the cartilage increases in density, apparently in an effort to compensate. As the disease progresses, bony growths or projections called osteophytes will form along the joint margins. Often in the joints of long bones, osteophyte formation takes on an appearance called "lipping" which can become quite pronounced. The articular cartilage can be completely eroded through exposing the bone surfaces. When this happens and motion continues, friction can cause the bone ends to become very smooth and polished, giving an "ivory" appearance. This is termed "eburnation" and occasionally can be seen in archaeological specimens. Other bone changes that can occur are roughening of the joint surfaces and deformity of bone ends through a remodeling process.

Table 2 shows some of the principal differences between degenerative joint disease and rheumatoid arthritis. Degenerative joint disease occurs in the aged, and there is no pronounced disability except in advanced cases. The incidence is equally divided between males and females.

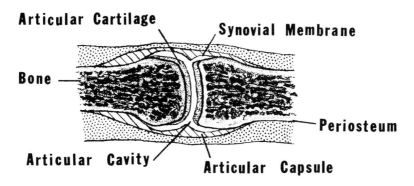

Fig. 1. Diagrammatic drawing of a normal diarthrosis. *Drawing by Alan Harn.*

Vertebral Osteophytosis

Degenerative joint disease of the vertebrae is called osteophytosis. There is no true synovial membrane so, technically, these intervertebral spaces are not true joints. A thick fibrocartilagenous membrane called the invertebral disc is located between the bodies of all vertebrae. The initial pathology in vertebral osteophytosis is the degeneration and later even the ultimate destruction of these discs. Osteophytes then form at the adjacent edges of the vertebrae, apparently in an effort to support the vertebral column, which has been made unstable by the destruction of the discs. The osteophytes can become quite large and, in projecting toward one another, will frequently fuse together, forming a bony bridging. In osteoarthritis of the other joints this fusion does not occur. There are all degrees of osteophytosis, ranging from very slight lipping of the margins of the vertebrae to complete bony fusion. The condition occurs most frequently in the lumbar region; the next most frequent location is the cervical area.

The principal conditions that should be differentiated from osteophytosis are healed compression fractures and ankylosing spondylitis. A healed compression fracture will occur (almost always) in only one area of the spine, and the collapse of the vertebrae can be diagnosed by x-ray examination (Plate 3,F). Ankylosing spondylitis, which will be discussed later, is the result of ossification of all spinal ligaments. Its appearance is that of a smooth, bony sheet-like covering over the surfaces of the vertebrae, which is somewhat different from the appearance of the roughened fused bony projections which occur in osteophytosis.

Osteoarthritis of the intervertebral joints between the articular processes may occur coincidentally because both osteoarthritis and vertebral osteophytosis are more prevalent in older ages.

Traumatic Arthritis

Traumatic arthritis is a joint disease initiated by trauma. This would include sprains, strains, fractures into the joint, and repeated injuries or unusual stress to a joint or joints. The resulting changes would be the same as those in degenerative joint disease. Archaeological diagnosis of traumatic arthritis would be difficult because one could not distinguish it from what it really is—degenerative bone disease. A presumed diagnosis could be made when there is evidence of an injury, such as a healed fracture or localized osteosclerosis, especially if only one joint is involved.

Rheumatoid Arthritis

The initial pathology in rheumatoid arthritis affects the soft tissues of the joint. At first the synovial membrane is inflamed. This causes swelling, thickening and scarring, which in turn produces severe deformities and limitation of motion. Pannus formation is a feature of rheumatoid arthritis. This consists of a proliferating nonspecific vascular connective tissue which forms on the surface of the synovial membrane. This can eventually

TABLE 2

DIFFERENTIAL DIAGNOSIS—ARTHRITIS

	DEGENERATIVE JOINT DISEASE	RHEUMATOID ARTHRITIS	ANKYLOSING SPONDYLITIS	VERTEBRAL OSTEOPHYTOSIS
SEX	1 male to 1 female	1 male to 4 females	More frequent in males 10 to 1	Initial pathology is degeneration of the intervertebral discs
AGE	Older ages; 40 plus 80% to 90% over 50	Younger ages; under 40	Fusion of vertebrae by ossification of ligaments	
PATH-OLOGY	Initially affects articular cartilage	Initially affects synovial membrane	Joints involved are: intervertebral, sacroiliac, costovertebral, articulations between the articular processes of the vertebrae, and sometimes the symphysis pubis	Lipping and formation of osteophytes on margins of vertebrae
	Destruction of cartilage	Chiefly disease of joint soft tissues		Osteophytes can fuse to give support to spinal column
	No early capsular changes	Edema and formation of scar tissue cause severe limitation of motion, ankylosis and deformities		Most frequent in lumbar and cervical vertebrae
	Osteophyte formation			
	Lipping			
	Deformity through remodeling	Pannus can cause destruction of cartilage and obliteration of joint		
	Eburnation (polishing due to friction of bone on bone)	Bone changes are osteoporosis, erosion near articular margins, and degenerative joint disease		
DISABIL-ITY	Rarely disabling	Moderate to severe		

result in a complete obliteration of the joint space and erosion of the articular cartilage. Significant bone changes will occur late and may take the form of degenerative joint disease; consequently in an advanced case of rheumatoid arthritis, with only the bone specimen, it might be impossible to distinguish between the two conditions: degenerative joint disease and rheumatoid arthritis. Osteoporosis of the bone near the affected joints is nearly always present. In addition, there may be some erosion of the bone beneath the articular cartilages and occasionally there may be bony ankylosis. Frequently, in advanced rheumatoid arthritis subluxation of the joints occurs; but this may not be apparent in archaeological specimens.

Clinically the diagnosis of rheumatoid arthritis is usually an easy matter. The archaeological diagnosis can be difficult to impossible. Plate 6,E shows a burial at Dickson Mounds, from which, because of the positioning of the burial *in situ* (knees flexed), one would suspect that the Indian suffered from a severe disabling rheumatoid arthritis. In addition there is some erosion of the bone ends of many of the joints near the articular surfaces (Plate 11,A). The same burial shows a mild degree of generalized degenerative joint disease.

Rheumatoid arthritis occurs almost four times more frequently in the female than in the male and is most common in the younger age group, usually those under 40. The disease not only affects many joints but also causes the victim to become quite ill. This illness plus the severe deformities and limitation of motion causes a moderate to severe disability.

Ankylosing Spondylitis

Ankylosing spondylitis has been thought to be a form of rheumatoid arthritis. Most authorities now consider it a distinct entity in itself. Other names for this condition are bamboo spine, poker spine, and Marie Strumpell's disease. The pathology consists of a calcification of ligaments. This includes the annulus fibrous (outer portion of the intervertebral disc), the longitudinal ligaments located anteriorly and posteriorly to the spinal column, the ligaments of the sacroiliac joints, and the ligaments associated with the articular processes of the vertebrae and the costovertebral joints. Occasionally there is a bony fusion of the symphysis pubis. Other joints of the body are not necessarily involved, but some degenerative joint disease might be present. There are all degrees of ankylosing spondylitis, ranging from involvement of the sacroiliac joints plus a few vertebrae to a complete bony fusion of the entire spine. Although osteophytes may appear in this disease, the bony connections between the joints usually have a smooth undulating surface which conforms somewhat to the contour of the spinal column. This has been described as having the appearance of being "poured on."

Ankylosing spondylitis occurs ten times more frequently in males than in females and produces moderate disability characterized by a kyphosis (bowing forward) and stiffness of the spine.

Infectious Arthritis

Infectious arthritis is inflammation of a joint caused by the presence of microorganisms. The pathological changes and the course of the disease in infectious arthritis depend on the type of microorganism involved, its virulence, and the resistance of the host. Because of these three factors, the condition can be classified as acute or chronic. The introduction of the causative organism into the joint can occur (1) by bloodstream transmission from a distant focus of infection, (2) by the extension of an infection (osteomyelitis) from a nearby bone, or (3) by direct introduction from a penetrating wound.

The most common microorganisms producing acute infectious arthritis are the staphylococci and the streptococci, and less frequently the meningococci, pneumococci, gonococci, and organisms of diphtheria, typhoid and others. When the organisms enter the joint space, they initially cause edema of the synovial membrane. Swelling and hyperemia occur and there is an increase of joint fluid. Occasionally this is the extent of the disease. The resistance of the host can cause the inflammation to subside. The joint may return to nearly its original state with little or no permanent gross bone changes. If the disease continues, the joint fluid will become purulent. This is called *pyogenic* or *suppurative* or *septic* arthritis. A substance is formed in the pus which has the ability to dissolve and destroy the cartilage.* Destruction of articular cartilage follows with an increase in the purulent joint fluid causing pressure which can lead to rupture of the joint capsule, creating abscesses in adjacent soft tissue or muscles. Further, the synovial membrane may be replaced by granulation and scar tissue. Projections of the pannus (see rheumatoid arthritis) will appear, leading to further destruction of the joint. Bone changes include osteoporosis, erosion, and osteitis—even osteomyelitis, which is most common in young children. At this stage a generalized septicemia (bloodstream infection) can appear, followed by death.

If the patient survives, then this acute arthritis becomes chronic. At first there is fibrous ankylosis, followed by deposition of cartilage and bone. The healing stage is usually characterized by the formation of a tremendous amount of bony regeneration, apparently an effort to give support to the destroyed joint. Archaeological specimens frequently show evidence of sinus tracts, suggesting that the abscess has been walled off by bone or scar tissue but purulent drainage continues throughout the life of the individual.

There are other types of infectious arthritis which can be classified as chronic because of the specific character of the infecting organism. One of the most common described in literature is chronic arthritis due to tubercle

---

*In infants and young children an unusual condition is sometimes seen, especially in the hip joint. Since almost the entire femoral head at that time is composed of cartilage, there can be very rapid disintegration of the entire head of the femur—followed by dislocation of the hip joint.

bacilli. This will be discussed in detail in a later chapter. The outstanding characteristic of tuberculosis is bone destruction with little or no bone regeneration. Treponema also can directly affect the joints, although a direct invasion of a joint by a treponema organism is rare. This will be discussed in a later chapter on specific diseases. Chronic arthritis can be caused also by many other kinds of infectious organisms, such as brucellosis and mycotic (fungus) infections, but these do not leave any specific bone changes which could justify an archaeological diagnosis.

There are other varieties of arthritis, only some of which have known causes. Two rather common conditions which should be mentioned here are rheumatic fever and gout.

In both instances a diagnosis by means of archaeological specimens is unlikely. Rheumatic fever is a transitory inflammation of the soft tissues of many joints. It leaves no residual bone pathology. Gout is a disease of unknown cause, where there is an increase in blood uric acid and a deposit of uric acid crystals in body tissues. The joints are the favorite location for these deposits particularly those of the lower extremities. The uric acid crystals cause a severe inflammation of the joint. These crystals later can be resorbed by the blood with no noticeable aftereffects. However, repeated attacks are the rule, and the joint or joints can become severely and permanently diseased, possibly with degenerative joint changes and bone erosion.

CHAPTER 5

INFLAMMATION OF BONE

Bone reacts to various irritants such as trauma, chemicals and infections in a similar manner. There is destruction of bone by bone resorption and formation of new bone by bone regeneration. We have already discussed the reaction of bone to trauma. This chapter will deal mostly with bone responses to infections. Inflammatory diseases of bone can be categorized as periostitis—inflammation of periosteum; osteitis—inflammation of the bone; and osteomyelitis—inflammation involving the marrow spaces. Seldom does one of these exist without the presence of one or both of the others.

Bone is one of the hardest substances in the body. It is tough and possesses elasticity. There are essentially two kinds of bone tissue: a dense tightly-packed ivory-like *compact* bone and a spongy or woven tissue called *cancellous* bone. Most of the bones of the body have a different amount of each of these bone elements. In the long bones the compact element is exterior and the spongy cancellous bone is interior, enclosing the marrow spaces. The periosteum covers all the exterior surfaces of the bone except where cartilage is attached. The interior lining of a bone, called the endosteum, lines the marrow cavity. In the bones of the cranium and face (membranous bones), there are two dense cortical layers called the inner and outer tables; in between is a section of cancellous bone called the *diploe*.

Periostitis

An inflammation confined principally to the periosteum can occur: by an extension into the bone from an adjacent soft-tissue infection; as part of a generalized disease such as syphilis, yaws, fungi infections, etc.; and by the involvement of the surface of the bone from an osteitis or osteomyelitis.

Localized periosteal bone regeneration as a response to overlying soft-tissue infection is rather common. The bone surface can appear irregular and there can be various degrees of nodulation and pitting. If the soft-tissue infection subsides, bone involvement can cease leaving telltale scars; or through remodeling, the bone can eventually return to nearly its original appearance.

Multiple or generalized periostitis is encountered rather frequently in prehistoric skeletal collections. In the Morse Site a Red Ocher burial F772-12 (Plate 13,A) had extensive periostitis. All the bones were involved except the skull. Two cases of multiple periostitis were found in the 1966 excavation at Dickson Mounds conducted by the Illinois State Museum. These two burials F34-284 and F34-294 are illustrated in Plate 14,B and Plate 15,D. Of approximately 400 skeletons examined from the Klunk Site there were nine cases of multiple periostitis. (The Klunk Site, located in Calhoun County, Illinois, was excavated by Gregory Perino for the Gilcrease Foundation.) Three distinct cultures were found in seven mounds: Hopewell, Archaic and Late Woodland. The pathology was reviewed by the author with the assistance of King Hunter, Department of Physical Anthropology, Indiana University. The tibiae were involved in all nine cases. Four of these cases are illustrated: C34-42 (Plate 13,C), C40-21 (Plate 15,A,B), C31-41 (Plate 14,C), and C36-40 (Plate 14,D).

Acute Osteomyelitis

Osteomyelitis is almost always caused by infection with a microorganism capable of producing pus (pyogenic). Osteomyelitis can occur by a direct extension of infection from the outside, as in the case of a compound fracture, or by hematogenous spread which means the organisms are carried from an infected area through the bloodstream to lodge in various bones and there set up multiple areas of osteomyelitis. Ninety percent of all cases of

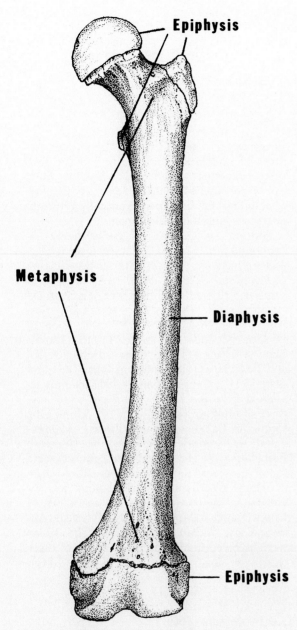

Fig. 2. Normal femur. *Drawing by Alan Harn.*

acute hematogenous osteomyelitis are due to staphylococci. The remaining 10 percent are due to pus-producing organisms, the streptococcus, pneumococcus, meningococcus, and occasionally to infection caused by the typhoid or colon bacilli.

The prognosis of acute infection depends on the tenacity of the infecting organism and the resistance of the intended victim. If conditions are unfavorable for the host, an acute osteomyelitis can be rapidly fatal. If the individual survives, the infection can become chronic. Chronic osteomyelitis can occur also in cases caused by organisms of lower virulence.

Chronic Osteomyelitis

Before the use of antibiotics, many cases of chronic osteomyelitis were characterized by multiple bone involvement. The victim would become chronically ill with many periods of remissions and exacerbations, and pus-draining sinuses which develop in the areas of infection would persist throughout life.

The pathology of osteomyelitis consists of bone destruction, abscess formation, and production of draining sinuses, and formation of involucra. Because of the nature of the blood supply to the bone, the hematogenous infection in the bone almost always starts in a marrow cavity, usually near the metaphysis (end of the bone). The infection may become localized in the bone end or spread throughout the marrow space; or, especially in young children, it may enter the joint space causing a septic arthritis. The reaction to the infectious organisms in the bone is similar to that occurring in other tissues. Initially there is an increase in the blood supply to the affected area, producing an edema and the formation of an exudate. At first the exudate will consist of a thin serous fluid; later due to the accumulation of debris and white blood cells, pus will develop. The pus may increase in volume and eventually, because of the increased pressure, rupture to the outside through the periosteum, forming a sinus tract. On rare occasions when the abscess becomes completely surrounded by bone, the causative organisms die, resulting in a Brodie's abscess. Such a condition probably would not be apparent in an archaeological specimen except by x-ray.

In osteomyelitis zones of dead bone which sometimes become separated from viable bone are called sequestra. Small sequestra, particularly those formed in cancellous bone, can be completely absorbed. Some will become dislodged and drain to the outside through a sinus tract. If a large sequestrum becomes entrapped, it can be removed only through surgery. Sometimes a sequestrum will consist of an entire shaft of a long bone. In a healing effort an involucrum may be formed. This is regeneration of new bone which sometimes will surround a sequestrum in an effort on the part of the body defenses to give support to the weakened bone. This involucrum, through a remodeling process, may take on the appearance and function of the bone shaft. Regeneration of bone can also be evidenced by the formation of variously sized nodules, located usually between areas of destruction, or by bone condensation, which can result in considerable thickening.

Chronic Non-suppurative Osteomyelitis

Non-suppurative sclerosing osteomyelitis of Garré is a rare bone disease characterized by osteosclerosis without the formation of pus. Clinically, it is an infectious painful condition which starts as an acute osteomyelitis. The predominant feature is the thickening of the affected bone. For the most part the disease is confined to a single bone, although multiple areas can be involved. Archaeologically, one would expect to find bone sclerosis with little or no evidence of abscesses or sinuses (see F34-293, Plate 17). The differential diagnosis must include healed fractures and bone tumors.

Granulomatous Lesions

Certain chronic infections, generally referred to as granulomas can cause an osteomyelitis which at times is indistinguishable from diseases caused by the common pyogenic organisms. Tuberculosis and treponema infections (syphilis and yaws) are the most common of these granulomata. These two diseases will be discussed in a later chapter. Sarcoid, a benign bone disease of unknown cause, produces small punched-out, cystic-like areas of rarefaction most commonly occurring in the phalanges of the hands and feet. A diagnosis of this disorder in archaeological material would be most unlikely but should be kept in mind when computing a differential diagnosis. Mycotic (fungus) infections can also be classed as granulomata. Mycotic disease of the bone is quite rare and usually occurs because of an extension of a nearby soft-tissue abscess into the bone. Occasionally mycotic infections can cause generalized bone osteitis and periostitis.

CHAPTER 6

TUMORS

A tumor can be defined as benign or malignant. A benign tumor, usually localized in one area, is slow-growing. If it can be completely removed surgically, it will not recur. A malignant tumor is much more serious; in the prehistoric Indian it was always fatal. It usually grows rapidly; it can invade and destroy surrounding tissues and organs; and it has the ability to metastasize; that is, small fragments of the tumor can break off and be carried to distant parts of the body through the blood or the lymphatics. These designations of benign and malignant do not always hold true, however. Some benign tumors can suddenly become malignant; and some tumors seem to fall into neither category but are "in-betweens."

A tumor can originate in the bone, such as osteoma or osteosarcoma; it can originate in nearby tissues and invade the bone by extension, such as a meningioma and some tendon-sheath tumors; or it can be a metastasis from any primary malignant tumor coming from any part of the body.

Sarcoma is a malignant tumor derived principally from connective tissue such as a fibrosarcoma (fibrous tissue), osteosarcoma (bone tissue), and chondrosarcoma (cartilage). Carcinoma is a malignant tumor derived from epithelial or glandular tissues, such as bronchogenic carcinoma and carcinoma of the prostate, thyroid, breast, etc.

A bone tumor, whether it is benign or metastatic, can cause: (1) bone destruction (osteolytic), (2) bone production (osteoplastic), or (3) a combination of both.

It is not the purpose here to discuss in detail every known tumor of the bone. A few of the more common tumors will be described. It will be a rarity, indeed, to accurately diagnose a specific tumor from dried bone specimens. The most important diagnostic tool used by pathologists is the microscopic appearance of the tumor cells; but this procedure is not available to the archaeologist.

TABLE 3
PRIMARY BONE TUMORS

ORIGIN	BENIGN	MALIGNANT
CARTILAGE	Chondroma Osteo chondroma	Chondrosarcoma
BONE	Osteoma Osteoid Osteoma Exostosis Bone Spurs	Osteosarcoma

CONNECTIVE TISSUE	Non-osteogenic
	  Fibroma
	Fibrous Cortical
	  Defect
	Giant-cell
	  Tumor
		Fibrosarcoma

VASCULAR	Hemangioma	Hemangiosarcoma

OTHER	Fibrous
	  Dysplasia
	Bone Cyst
	Aneurysmal
	  Bone Cyst
	Eosiniphilic
	  Granuloma
		Ewing's Sarcoma
		Multiple Myeloma

Benign Tumors

Osteochondroma is one of the most common of the benign tumors. It consists of an overgrowth of cartilage and bone—only the bony portion remains in the archaeological specimen. These tumors can be solitary or multiple and occur more often in the ends of the long bones (metaphyses). They are thought to be congenital; but because of their slow growth, they are not usually discovered until late childhood. Occasionally, malignant changes will develop.

A *chondroma* can occur in any bone pre-formed by cartilage. This includes all bones except the vault of the cranium and the upper face. These tumors can be single or multiple and can arise externally or internally to a bone. If there is no ossification of the cartilage, which can occur, archaeological specimens will show only a bone defect with little or no surrounding bone condensation. The most favored sites of the chondromas are the fingers, toes, pelvis, sternum and ribs.

An *osteoma* is found almost always in the bones of the cranium and jaw. It consists of an overgrowth of osseous tissue, slow growing and rarely causing trouble (Plate 19,A). Its borders are sharply defined, as demonstrated in an x-ray (Plate 19,A). An osteoma could be confused with the bone sclerosis following trauma, healed fractures, and *osteoid osteoma*. An x-ray of an osteoid osteoma will typically show a small area of rarefaction located in the cortex or spongy portion of a long bone surrounded by moderately thick bone condensation. Sometimes this bone condensation is very large causing a prominent swelling of the bone shaft.

Small circular bony projections are a common occurrence, mostly located on the bones of the cranium. These small "osteomata" can be dome-shaped or flattened, and sometimes they are stemmed, giving the appearance of tiny mushrooms (Plate 19,D). Another group of bone growths are called *exostoses* or *bony spurs*. Most of these are probably a response to trauma or adjacent infection. Ear *exostoses* are bony growths located in the external auditory canal. Sometimes they are so numerous or large as to cause occlusion. This condition is rather rare but is more frequent in certain races or groups of people (Hrdlicka 1935): rare in African Negroes and Europeans and more common in Polynesians and American Indian groups. Don Dickson was the first to point out the frequent occurrence of ear exostoses in the Illinois Hopewellian crania (Adis-Castro and Neumann 1948). (See Plate 18,D.) It has been suggested that some sort of trauma would stimulate the appearance of these ear tumors. One possibility may be the wearing of heavy ear ornaments. The Hopewell Indians wore large ear-spools, but so did other cultures where the incidence of ear exostoses is much less.

A *giant-cell tumor* has been classified as a benign primary bone tumor. However, the term *benign* is misleading; for the prognosis is unfavorable. Recovery does not occur without surgery, and, even with surgery, recurrences are common. In addition a certain number are or will become malignant and will metastasize. This tumor, usually located in the epiphyseal portion of a long bone, is found most frequently in individuals between the ages of 20 to 40. The name is derived from the fact that a microscopic section shows the presence of many multinuclear giant cells, not evident, of course, in archaeological specimens. Pathologically the tumor causes extensive destruction of bone (osteolytic) with little or no new bone formation. The x-ray shows an area of rarefaction at the end of a bone with thinning of the cortex and sometimes an expansion of the bone end. In advanced cases the boundaries may be represented by a thin shell of bone, oftentimes perforated, permitting the tumor to extend itself into the soft tissues. Giant-cell tumors are rare. The diagnosis is difficult to impossible in dried bones. The conditions that can mimic this tumor include: bone cyst, aneurysmal bone cyst, hemangioma, fibrous dysplasia, ossifying and nonossifying fibroma and many of the bone sarcomas.

A *non-osteogenic fibroma*, most frequent in young persons, is usually a single lesion occurring near the end of the diaphysis of a long bone. On the x-ray it appears as an area of rarefaction with irregular margins. It would be difficult to differentiate non-osteogenic fibroma from a solitary lesion of a fibrous dysplasia. Another name for this condition is *non-ossifying fibroma* of bone. A *fibrous cortical defect* is a term given to a rather common small osseous defect confined to the cortex of a long bone. It occurs in very young children and is almost always clinically silent—usually being discovered by x-rays taken for some other reason. Its favorite location is the distal metaphysis of a femur. Usually the lesion remains small and may disappear, but occasionally it persists and becomes quite large.

According to Jaffe (1958, Chapter 6), "When it does this, the lesion ceases to be a mere fibrous cortical defect and becomes what we call a non-ossifying fibroma of bone."

A *hemangioma* is found frequently in vertebrae, less frequently in the bones of the cranium, and rarely in other bones. In a vertebra, it is usually small and is restricted to the body. It seldom causes symptoms. Although the tumor can be multiple, i.e., occur in more than one vertebra, it will not cross the intervertebral disc and invade an adjoining vertebra. Occasionally it occupies an entire vertebral body. Clinically, this can result in pressure on the spinal cord. Archaeologically, a hemangioma will give the appearance of an irregularly shaped cyst-like hole. In the skull the hemangioma can appear on the x-ray to be multilocular and to portray a "sunray" appearance with longitudinal spicules radiating from the center to the outer edges. The cranial tumor originates in the diploic spaces. It can erode through either table but usually will cause only a slight bulging of the outer table.

A *meningioma* is not a primary bone tumor. It is mentioned here because it could be confused, archaeologically but probably not clinically, with a hemangioma. Originating in the covering of the brain, it may erode into a cranial bone, causing at least a minimal perforation. A major characteristic is the development of a great deal of hyperostosis which can take on the pattern of radiating bony spicules. A much-quoted prehistoric case was found in Peru in the Inca ruins of Paucarcancha (MacCurdy 1923). The first diagnosis was osteosarcoma. Later, several experts changed this impression to meningioma (Zariquiey 1958).

Fibrous dysplasia, a process where areas of bone are replaced by fibrous tissue, can exist in two forms: the multiple or polyostotic lesion which is rare; and the more common solitary or monostotic lesion, confined to one bone. The disease predominates in females (at least 2 to 1) and when only one bone is affected, the most usual location is the femur, tibia, rib or face. The etiology is unknown. Whether the condition can be classified as a tumor is not certain. It has been suggested that the disease is an endocrine disturbance, but this has not been proven (Moldawer and Rabin 1966). Frequently it is unilateral (confined to one side of the body). Fractures and deformities are prominent features. In 1930 a University of Chicago field party, working in Fulton County, Illinois, excavated the skeleton of a badly crippled 35-year-old male belonging to the Mississippian culture. This find was reported in detail by Dr. H. S. Denninger (1931), and later by Cole and Deuel (1937). The pathology consisted of multiple cysts with resulting deformities confined to the left side of the body. The original diagnosis proposed by Dr. Denninger was "osteitis fibrosa." When Dr. Denninger's article was reprinted as Chapter 28 in *Diseases in Antiquity* (Brothwell and Sandison 1967), the editors suggested that the diagnosis should be changed to *fibrous dysplasia*. We now know that *osteitis fibrosa cystica* is a generalized disease caused by overactivity of the parathyroid glands.

A *solitary bone cyst* is probably not a true tumor. It occurs in children from the ages of three to twenty. When it persists in the adult, all growth ceases and it is called a *latent cyst*. It is almost always located in the upper metaphyses of the humerus, femur or tibia, rarely occurring in other bones. The cyst, appearing as a hole or defect in the bone caused by bone resorption, is lined with a thin intact layer of cortical bone. On the x-ray film its shape appears to be circular with smooth borders or multilocular with irregular walls. Although there may be localized widening of the bone, the "shell" of bone surrounding the cyst remains intact. In the case of fracture, which is common in the weakened area, there is periosteal thickening, a part of the repair process. In the young child, the cyst is always found in the metaphysis near the epiphysis. In older children and adults, the cyst may be located in the shaft of the long bone. This apparent movement of the cyst down the shaft occurs because the lesion became inactive while there is still some bone growth at the epiphyseal ends. A solitary cyst may cause no clinical symptoms unless a fracture occurs. Sometimes the cyst will improve or heal when the fracture undergoes repair. An archaeological differential diagnosis would include: solitary fibrous dysplasia, fibrous cortical defect, non-ossifying fibroma, aneurysmal bone cyst and a single lesion of eosinophilic granuloma.

An *aneurysmal bone cyst* is usually encountered in the shaft of a long bone or in a vertebra. Rarely is it found in other locations such as the pelvis and the cranium. When it involves a long bone, it is likely to be on one side of the bone shaft. When it is in a vertebra, it may result in a collapse. It gets its name from the appearance of the x-ray and the fact that the cyst is filled with blood. A typical x-ray of the lesion in a long bone will show a ballooned-out area of rarefaction with a thin outer border, causing an eccentrically located bulging of the bone and having the appearance of being multilocular. This multilocular effect can persist in dried bone specimens because part of the borders of the spaces within the cyst contain thin layers of bone.

Eosinophilic granuloma, Letterer-Siwe disease and Schuller-Christian disease, are considered by most authorities to be different manifestations of the same condition. Another name applied to all of these conditions is *histiocytosis* X. The basic pathology is a granulomatous proliferation of reticulum cells (Moseley 1963:161; Ritvo 1955:448; Collins 1966:174; and Luck 1950:410). When this proliferation involves bone, the result is a localized destruction of the bone by the granulomatous tissue. There is a minimal amount of bone condensation surrounding the lesions. Letterer-Siwe and Schuller-Christian diseases attack many other systems of the body beside the skeleton—especially the lungs—and the mortality rate is high. *Eosinophilic granuloma* rarely, if ever, causes death. It presumably affects bone only, although there has been some recent disagreement on this point (Collins 1966:180). The solitary or multiple lesions, occurring in both flat and long bones, appear in infants, children and very young adults. Spontaneous resolution is common. The nature and etiology of histiocytosis X is unknown. Whether it is a tumor, infection or something else has not yet been determined.

Malignant

Among the most difficult problems in clinical medicine is that of accurately diagnosing the specific type of primary malignant bone tumor and, including the examination of pathological specimens, to differentiate between the benign and the malignant. Archaeologically, these difficulties are multiplied.

Probably the most frequent primary bone tumor is *osteosarcoma*. This tumor has a higher incidence in males and is usually found within the ages of 10 to 25. The long bones are most frequently involved, especially the femur. These tumors can be almost totally destructive with little or no new bone formation—in which case they are called "osteolytic osteosarcoma"—or there can be a great deal of ossification. These are termed "sclerosing osteosarcoma." Many tumors have a variable amount of both ossification and destruction.

A *chondrosarcoma* is a malignant tumor of cartilage. It can either be "central"—arising from the interior of a bone, or "secondary"—evolving from a preexisting chondroma. Chondrosarcomas can contain some bone, and also calcified material in an irregular pattern, since many of them contain dystrophic zones of calcification. Archaeologically, one would see only the destruction caused by the cartilage tumor invasion plus any new bone that might have formed; consequently the probability of making a diagnosis would be very remote. A *fibrosarcoma* is entirely osteolytic and contains no new bone. A *hemangiosarcoma*, a malignant tumor originating from vascular tissue within a bone, is very rare. A benign hemangioma never becomes malignant. The predominant feature is bone destruction. *Ewing's sarcoma* is a highly malignant bone tumor of children and young adults which originates from the medullary space, causing expansion of the bone. Ewing's tumor produces severe bone destruction but has no power in itself to produce bone. Some bone condensation occurs as a reactive process. Successive reactive periosteal new-bone formation can give an "onion peel" appearance on the x-ray. This tumor is most frequently found in the long bones and the flat bones of the pelvis. One peculiarity is that the lesion is "always" more extensive than indicated by the x-ray and the gross specimen. Frequently autopsy reveals extensive tumor infestation throughout the entire skeleton. This finding is generally considered not to be evidence of metastatic spread but that simultaneous involvement of many bones is characteristic of this deadly disease.

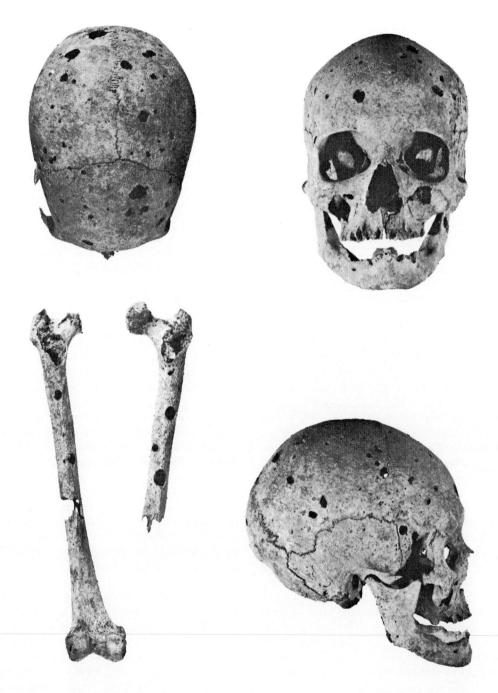

Fig. 3. Both femora and three views of skull are indicative of multiple myeloma. Kane Site, Madison County, Illinois. *Photograph, courtesy of Dr. Sheilagh Brooks and the Museum of Northern Arizona.*

Primary bone tumors metastasize freely to all tissues and organs of the body but rarely metastasize to bone. One of the most frequent locations for the deposit of these metastases is the lungs. These deposits could be, in part, osseous tissue and therefore could become an archaeological find. The author is unaware of any such discovery, probably because it would necessitate a very careful excavation by an excavator who was aware of the possibility. There have been many recoveries of kidney stones by archaeologists (Plate 32,A, B), and metastatic bone nodules would be somewhat similar, although of much rarer occurrence.

A bone-proliferating osteosarcoma could be mistaken for a healed fracture with heavy callus formation. A differential point would be that the tumor would cause a total disruption of normal bone structure while the fracture, through remodeling, would result in the restoration of a marrow space and bone cortex.

Multiple myeloma is a widespread and fatal malignant tumor that originates in the bone marrow. It almost always occurs in individuals over 40 and more frequently in those between the ages of 50 to 70. The bone changes are characterized by a pronounced generalized osteoporosis and by the presence of many sharply demarcated "punched-out" areas of lysis of various sizes, disseminated throughout the skeleton. Grossly, the holes appear as though they had been made by an instrument such as a paper punch. The edges show no evidence of any osteoblastic activity. All bones in the body can be involved, but especially the skull, ribs, spine, and long bones. In the shoulder, sometimes only the outer end of the clavicle and the acromion will be affected; occasionally a fibula will show the disease while the tibia in the same leg will not. Solitary lesions have been reported, but some of these have been shown to be precursors of dissemination. Pathological fractures, caused by coalesence of the tumors, are common (Plate 32,D,E,F).

Brooks and Melbye (1967) report a case of multiple myeloma from the Kane Site, near St. Louis. This is a female about 40 years of age (Mississississippian). Scattered throughout most of the skeleton are punched-out perforations from 2 to 17 mm. in diameter (Fig. 3).

Metastases to the Skeleton

Primary malignant bone tumors are usually single, while secondary (metastatic) tumors are usually multiple. The skeleton is very frequently invaded by metastatic disease. Carcinomas will metastasize to bone more than sarcomas. In certain carcinomas such as prostate, thyroid, breast and lung, the incidence of bone metastases can be as high as 80 percent. A primary bone tumor occurs in young people, usually those under 40, while most secondary osseous tumors appear after the age of 40. Statistically, secondary tumors are more frequent than primary malignant tumors, but this would not be applicable to prehistoric Indians because of their shorter life expectancy. All bones of the skeletons are subject to metastases, but those most frequently affected are the skull, ribs, vertebra, pelvis and femora.

Secondary tumors of bone can be *osteolytic* (bone destruction), *osteoplastic* (bone proliferation), or a combination of both. Most malignancies are osteolytic and occasionally a large portion of a bone can be entirely destroyed. Most of the metastases originating from carcinoma of the prostate are osteoplastic, as are some from carcinoma of the breast and bronchogenic (lung) carcinoma. These osteoplastic lesions will show increased bone density by x-ray and by cross-section examination. The tumor itself does not produce bone, but it does have the property of stimulating bone production by the bone osteoblasts.

One difficult problem in dealing with skeletal material is to differentiate between an osteolytic metastatic tumor and a multiple myeloma. Generally, a multiple myeloma would be expected to be more widely distributed.

CHAPTER 7

ANOMALIES

This chapter will consider a few of the many abnormal changes found in the skeleton which would not be appropriate for inclusion in any of the other chapters in this book. They are: (1) changes due to endocrine disturbances; (2) changes caused by nutritional deficiencies; (3) lesions associated with blood disorders; (4) congenital abnormalities; and (5) miscellaneous defects.

Endocrine Disturbances
The endocrine glands secrete chemical substances, called hormones, which maintain a normal status in many of the body functions. When any endocrine gland malfunctions, that is, secretes too much or too little, disturbances and changes occur. The interreaction and interdependence of these ductless glands often make it difficult to determine which gland causes what abnormality. The glands that more commonly create abnormal changes in the skeleton are: pituitary, adrenal, thyroid, parathyroid and the gonads.

The *pituitary* gland, located at the base of the brain in a fossa of the sella turcica, is known to secrete many different hormones, the function of most of which is not clearly understood. Two of these hormones cause pronounced bone changes. If excessive secretion of a growth hormone occurs prior to the ossification of the epiphyses, the result is *giantism*. If the excess production of this growth hormone occurs in the adult, the result is *acromegaly*. The skeleton of a pituitary giant is usually of normal proportions unless there is some superimposed acromegaly. Pituitary giants are rare because tumors of the anterior lobe of the pituitary gland, which bring about oversecretion, are infrequent in young people. Pituitary giants can be confused with normal large individuals.

Numerous and bizarre changes in the skeleton occur in the acromegalic. These changes will vary widely, depending on the severity of the disease and the age of the occurrence. Characteristic features of the skeleton include:
(1) Thickening and enlargement of all bones of the skull.
(2) A disproportionate broadening and elongation of the lower jaw, causing a protrusion (prognathism).
(3) The nasal sinuses are greatly expanded.
(4) The teeth become separated and there is malocclusion.
(5) All bones of the postcranial skeleton become larger.
(6) There is elongation of the bones of the hands and feet with tufting of the terminal phalanges.
(7) The bodies of the lower cervical and thoracic vertebrae become enlarged dorsally and laterally.
Decrease in the secretion of this growth hormone will result in a pituitary dwarf. The skeletal proportions may remain those of an infant or child, depending on the time of the onset of the disease. This accounts for the head being large. In addition there is a retardation of tooth eruption and failure of, or delay in, ossification of the epiphyseal plates.

Another hormone secreted by the anterior lobe of the pituitary is called ACTH (adrenocorticotropin), thought to originate in the basophilic cells. Overactivity or tumor of these cells results in excessive secretion of ACTH. ACTH regulates the production of cortisone, a hormone produced by the cortex of the *adrenal* gland. Too much ACTH means too much cortisone, which can cause a disturbance of bone metabolism resulting in an insufficient amount of bone martix. This is linked with protein formation and the bone will contain less minerals. The end result is severe osteoporosis. This disease is called *Cushing's syndrome*. Another and probably more common cause of Cushing's syndrome, independent of the pituitary gland, is hyperfunction of the adrenal cortex caused by tumor or hyperplasia. All bones can be involved, but the spine, pelvis and skull may be more seriously affected. Frequent pathological fractures are the rule. An identical condition can occur in individuals who have been on corticosteroid therapy for long periods. The gonads secrete sex hormones that are believed to be antagonistic to the osteoporotic effect of the corticosteroids. As long as both of these hormones are of normal quantities, bone metabolism is normal. In old age the hormone of the cortex of the adrenal remains at a normal level but there is a decrease in sex hormones, causing an imbalance in favor of the corticosteroids. This is thought to be the cause of senile osteoporosis, but this theory is not universally accepted. Senile osteoporosis occurs earlier and more frequently in the female.

A decrease or absence of the secretion of the hormone of the *thyroid gland* may cause bony changes depending on the onset of deficiency. Hypothyroidism in the adult results in no particular changes in the bones. If the disease occurs at birth, or because of a congenital absence of the thyroid, the result is a *cretin*. If the deficiency begins in infancy or childhood, the condition is termed *infantile myxedema*. The principal feature is dwarfing. As in the pituitary dwarf, the proportions and appearance of the skeleton will depend on the severity and the time of onset. Clinically the pituitary dwarf is of normal mentality while the cretin is mentally retarded.

A tumor or hyperactivity of the *parathyroid glands* results in *osteitis fibrosa cystica*. The basic pathology is the secretion of an excessive amount of calcium and phosphorus by the kidneys, resulting in a demineralization of the skeleton. The gross appearance of dried bones would be a generalized osteoporosis not only because of less mineral content but also a decrease in bone matrix. In addition, there will be many variously sized areas where there is an absence of bone tissues. These are the end results of the cysts and brown tumors seen in the fresh bone specimens and x-rays. X-rays of the bones will show a decrease in density and the scattered cysts. X-rays of the phalanges of the fingers are believed by some to be of great diagnostic value. The middle phalanges

will show a "lace-like" decalcification of the cortex with subperiosteal resorption of bone. The treatment of this condition is surgical removal of the parathyroid tumor. Pathological fractures and bending deformities are frequent.

Nutritional Deficiencies

The body needs certain foods, such as proteins, carbohydrates, fats and minerals plus essential chemicals called vitamins. A deficiency in all (famine) or any one of these can cause changes in the skeleton, the most frequent being osteoporosis and an interference of normal growth. It is unlikely that a diagnosis of a specific food deficiency could be made with any degree of certainty from archaeological specimens—with the possible exception of *rickets*, caused by lack of vitamin D, and *scurvy*, a vitamin C deficiency.

Vitamin D is necessary for the absorption of calcium from the intestine. An inadequate supply of vitamin D causes *rickets* in infancy and childhood during the bone-growing period and *osteomalacia* in the adult. This vitamin can come from two sources: foods such as fish, meat, egg yolk and oysters, and the action of sunlight on the skin.

The pathology of rickets is principally a disturbance of bone growth and a demineralization of the skeleton: the normal bone matrix is produced but is not properly calcified, and the bones become soft and pliable. Bending deformities occur especially in weight-bearing areas—bowlegs, chest deformities, contracted pelvis and scoliosis. These may persist after healing. A beading enlargement of the ribs at the costal-sternal junction is a feature of active rickets. This beading, due to overgrowth of uncalcified osteoid tissue, probably would be lost in dried bone; but a flaring of the anterior ends of the ribs may persist. There could be an enlargement of the ends of the long bones because of a buildup of noncalcified osteoid tissue. Transverse lines, thought to be the result of incomplete fractures, may occur in the shafts of the long bones (Looser zones). The gross and x-ray appearance of the dried bone specimens would depend on the stage of the disease at the time of death—whether active, healed or healing.

In rickets and osteomalacia there may follow a hyperfunction of the parathyroid glands, apparently in an effort to mobilize calcium from the bones. This factor is responsible for producing superimposed bone lesions, similar to those of hyperparathyroidism. Bone changes, somewhat similar to those occurring in rickets and osteomalacia, may take place in the following:

(1) Certain chronic kidney disorders resulting in "renal rickets." The mechanism for this is not clearly understood. Somehow the dietary calcium and also probably the phosphorus are not available for adequate bone metabolism.

(2) Deficiency of calcium and/or phosphorus in the diet.

(3) Idiopathic hypercalciuria—over-excretion of calcium by the kidneys, the cause of which is unknown.

(4) Vitamin D resistance—an inherited (?) disorder in which the body is unable to utilize vitamin D.

Since vitamin C is found in fruit, leafy vegetables, peppers, beans, pumpkins, etc., it is conceivable that scurvy might have developed in prehistoric populations during long winters. However, according to Collins (1966: 101), the signs of the disease do not appear until many months after the individual stops ingesting the vitamin.

Bone changes in scurvy are reversible when the disease heals. If death should occur before healing is complete, the archaeologist might suspect its presence especially if many individuals in the same excavation unit showed the same evidences. Bone changes during the course of scurvy can include:

(1) Generalized deossification of the skeleton. The cortices may become "paper thin." This is believed to be caused mostly by immobility due to pain.

(2) Subperiosteal hemorrhages. The blood appearing beneath the periosteum can be absorbed or may clot. The clot can become a callus. When healing is complete, the callus can be resorbed through remodeling and the bone can return to its original shape. Hemorrhages can also occur into the metaphyses.

(3) Bleeding will occur in the bone tissue surrounding the teeth, causing erosion and necrosis. The teeth become loosened and may be lost.

(4) In the growing skeleton, pronounced changes will appear at the epiphyseal lines and at the metaphyses. This is due to the disturbance in bone formation in which the production of bone is retarded or ceases, but the resorption proceeds at the regular rate. Due to this weakening, fractures at the bone ends and epiphyseal separations are common.

Cribra orbitalis, mentioned in Chapter 1, is thought to be a porosis of the bones of the orbit with numerous small pits or holes. The same condition will occur in other areas of the skull (Plate 23,F). Most cases of this abnormality demonstrate that the bones are far from being porotic. They are quite dense with some overgrowth of regenerated bone surrounding the tiny pits. Possibly these overgrowths represent healed lesions which at one time may have shown hyperporosis caused by a period of malnutrition or illness. This condition is frequent whenever one examines a large collection of excavated skeletons.

Growth arrest lines (Harris's lines) are thin transverse lines of increased density usually spaced at irregular intervals at the ends of some of the long bones. These linear areas of increased calcification are visible on x-rays and microscopic sections and sometimes can be seen on the gross specimen, especially if the bone is split longitudinally. They are thought to be the results of arrested growth caused by nutritional disturbance or some acute illness that lasts at least ten days (Collins 1966:37). Calvin Wells (1967) suggests that the average number of these transverse lines in a specific skeleton collection might give an indication of "an index of morbidity." It is emphasized that it is not possible to tell the nature of the illness that produces a Harris's line. Wells further suggests that the distance of any particular line from the end of the bone represents the diaphyseal length of the bone at the time of the illness; from this, then, it is possible to estimate the age of the child at that time. These lines may be seen microscopically before x-ray evidence appears

(Collins 1966) and the x-ray may show lines which may not yet be visible grossly (Wells 1967). In the 1968 annual meeting of the American Association of Physical Anthropologists, Patricia Schwager, University of Pennsylvania, presented a study of 201 children of whom 199 have "transverse" tibial lines. The adult stature of these children showed no difference between those having many lines and those having only a few. This means that the presently accepted name "arrested growth" is suspect (Garn and Schwager 1967). It may be that the growth was temporarily interrupted and later accelerated with no effect on the final height.

In some primitive societies today, only a small percentage of children survive for more than a few years. The cause of this is believed to be poor nutrition due to feeding problems and intestinal infections due to poor sanitation. Whenever these conditions are improved in developing countries, the infant mortality rate declines sharply. The appearance of the dried skeletons of these modern young children has never been documented. The same conditions of deprivation existed in most of the prehistoric societies of the Midwest. The bones of many of these children have been examined or are awaiting examination. It would be expected that bone abnormalities found in these infants and young children would not have been caused by a single clinical entity but would have resulted from a combination of tragedies such as illness, nutritional deficiency, anemia, etc.

Examination of over 400 skeletons from the Klunk Site by King Hunter revealed that over 20 percent were under the age of two, and that nearly all of these and many of the older children showed various degrees of osteoporosis. Some showed swelling of bone ends, a few had growth-arrest lines and at least six had obliteration or partial loss of the medullary spaces. Of the 101 individuals at the Klunk Site belonging to the Archaic culture, 23 percent died before the age of two and 48 percent before the age of nine. Of the 294 Hopewellians, 14 percent died before age two and 26 percent before age nine. Of the 64 Late Woodland burials at Klunk, 14 percent died before age two and an additional 7 percent, making a total of 21 percent, before age

nine. Comparison of these three cultures is not justified, as some prehistoric groups are known to not bury all their children in mounds with the adults, but elsewhere, such as beneath house floors or in cemeteries. If this occurred at Klunk, then the child mortality rate would be yet higher. Personal communication with Gregory Perino revealed that some of the Woodland mounds at the Klunk Site contained no infants.

Blood Disorders

Anemias may cause significant bone changes, some of which might be considered specific. The changes are thought to be caused by two factors: (1) hyperplasia of all elements of the bone marrow in an effort to produce more red blood cells to compensate for those being lost, and (2) a spasm or thrombosis of the blood vessel supply to the bones. The resulting infarction interferes with bone nutrition and may result in areas of necrosis. The extent and location of bone pathology will depend on the severity, type, and duration of the anemia.

Some of the anemias that can be associated with bone disease (Karsner 1955; Moseley 1963; Perou 1964) are:

(1) *Iron deficiency anemia.* Lack of iron in the diet or, in the case of the infant, the mother's diet. Excessive need because of unusually rapid growth of the child. Chronic hemorrhage such as might occur in hookworm infestation, scurvy, etc.

(2) *Hemolytic anemia of the newborn (erythroblastosis fetalis).* This occurs when the mother's blood is Rh negative and the fetal blood is Rh positive. The mother's blood will produce a defense antibody which unfortunately crosses the placenta, resulting in destruction (hemolysis) of the fetal red blood cells.

(3) *Congenital hemolytic jaundice.* This is an inherited increased fragility of the red blood cells.

(4) *Sickle-cell disease.* This anemia is inherited, confined almost entirely to Negroes, and is characterized by abnormally shaped red cells.

(5) *Thalassemia (Mediterranean anemia),* This inherited condition until recently was considered limited to Mediterranean people

and their descendants but has been reported in American Indians and Negroes. There are several recognized classifications of this disease. It may be mild (thalassemia minor) or severe (thalassemia major). Probably the most severe bone lesions are encountered in the thalassemias.

Symmetrical osteoporosis of the skull, the most important bone lesion associated with anemia, occurs in various degrees of severity, being more pronounced in Mediterranean anemia. There is an overgrowth of the marrow in the skull, resulting in widening of the diploic space. The outer table is thinned and sometimes undergoes complete atrophy. Often the coarsened trabeculae will be arranged perpendicularly to the inner table, creating a "hair-on-end" appearance in the x-ray, also plainly visible on the gross cross section. The frontal bone is the most frequent location, but all bones of the skull can be involved. In severe instances the hyperplastic enlargement of the maxillary, sphenoidal and temporal bones may impede or prevent the formation of paranasal sinuses. *Porotic hyperostosis* is a more appropriate term for this condition (Angel 1967). Attempts to relate porotic hyperostosis to cribra orbitalis have not been very convincing.

Changes in the postcranial skeleton will occur, especially in sickle-cell disease and the thalassemias, and less frequently in iron-deficiency anemia. There can be osteoporosis and a thinning of the cortex due to hyperplasia of the bone marrow. Occasionally new bone may form on the inner aspect of the cortex, resulting in a narrowing of the medullary spaces. Profound changes can occur, especially in sickle-cell anemia, due to necrosis caused by thrombosis or spasm of the blood vessels supplying the bones. In dried bone specimens, these lesions, at times, can simulate and be indistinguishable from periostitis and even osteomyelitis (Moseley 1963 and 1966; Angel 1967).

Hemophilia is an inherited defect of blood coagulation characterized by excessive bleeding. Most cases of hemophilia are sex-linked and confined to males (Moseley 1963:46). The outstanding pathology is bleeding into the joints, which may result in cartilage destruc-

tion, bone erosion, cyst formation and degenerative changes including loss of joint space, irregularity of bone ends and osteophyte production. Subperiosteal hemorrhage is an uncommon feature of this condition.

Leukemia is a fatal disease which could be considered analogous to a malignancy (cancer) of white blood cells. It can be acute or chronic. Most bone changes occur in the acute form in children. They include: osteolytic lesions, periosteal elevation, osteosclerosis and a transverse line of rarefaction at the ends of some long bones—as seen by x-ray. The findings are not extensive and certainly, in dried bone specimens, would not be specific or diagnostic.

Myelosclerosis is a disorder thought by many to be related to leukemia. There is anemia and fibrotic or sclerotic changes in the bone marrow (Moseley 1963). About a third of the cases show bone lesions, such as generalized or patchy osteosclerosis and there may be a narrowing of the medullary spaces by formation of new bone on the inner surfaces of the cortices.

Congenital Defects

Almost every skeleton will have one or more minor deviations from normal. The majority of these apparent congenital abnormalities are inconsequential. They cause no disability and have no selective factor that might be considered advantageous or detrimental for survival. In most cases the individual is not aware of the existence of these defects. The definition of congenital is "existing at time of birth." Most congenital defects are considered inherited or "inborn," as is obviously the case with polydactylism (extra digits). On the other hand a congenital birth injury is acquired as opposed to being inborn (genetic). In some abnormalities it is not known whether they are inherited, acquired by environmental influences, or a combination of both. An example of the latter would be the increased susceptibility to an infectious disease. An attempt will be made to describe some of the congenital defects that have been found in archaeological specimens.

Deviations in head shape can be caused by: (1) premature closure of a specific suture, thus stopping growth in the area of that suture but permitting growth at other suture lines, and (2) simply the overgrowth of one area of the skull. (See Pancoast et al., 1940; Brothwell 1963 and 1967; Hohenthal and Brooks 1960.)

Scaphocephaly (boat- or keel-shaped skull) is a result of a premature closure of the *sagittal* suture. The skull vault is long and narrow with some medial ridging.

Oxycephaly (tower skull) will follow an early ossification of the transverse (coronal and lambdoid) sutures. There is an increase in height (pointed head) and often width of the skull. There is a good deal of variation in the shape, depending on the extent of involvement of the sutures. Turricephaly and acrocephaly are other names for this defect.

Trigonocephaly (triangle-shaped skull) is a pointed forehead following a premature synostosis of the *metopic* suture. Normally, this suture divides the frontal bone into halves and will close before the age of two. If it closes prior to this time, there may be a narrowed frontal bone with bulging.

Plagiocephaly is an asymmetrical vault which makes the skull appear to be normally developed on one side and underdeveloped on the other, or one side more developed anteriorly and the other side posteriorly.

Microcephaly (small head) probably has nothing to do with premature suture closures. Many microcephalics are idiots. Two examples of microcephalia were found in a Late Woodland mound at the Riviera aux Vase Site, Macomb County, Michigan. One of these is shown in Plate 24,A.

Hydrocephaly (large head) is the result of increased intracranial pressure caused by infection, tumor or injury. It may be present at the time of birth but most are postnatal. A pronounced hydrocepahlic is severely handicapped and long survival is unlikely. The increased pressure leads to enlargement of the head. There may be some separation of the bones at the suture lines and the cranial bones become very thin (Plate 24,B).

Malformations associated with premature craniostenoses should not be confused with genetic variation, such as may occur in racial differences (Neumann 1952 and 1961), with those artificially produced (binding or the cradleboard), or with postmortem changes due mostly to earth pressure. It has been suggested that a premature closure of a suture may be a symptom and not the cause. It may be a secondary characteristic produced as a result of a primary genetic bone factor (Bennett 1967).

Accessory skull bones are common. The metopic suture may persist throughout life, dividing the frontal bone bilaterally into halves. An extra suture may cross the upper portion of the occipital bone, forming a triangle-shaped *inca* bone. *Wormian* or sutural bones are extremely frequent. Brothwell (1963) reports that the percentage frequency of Wormian bones in different population groups varies from 25 percent in the Eskimo up to 80.32 percent in the Chinese. A rather uncommon occurrence is the presence of an anomalous suture dividing the zygomatic process forming the *os japonicum* (Anderson 1962). Kenneth Bennett (1965) suggests that Wormian bones "are not under direct genetic control, but instead represent secondary sutural characteristics which are brought about by stress." This would explain the high incidence of Wormian bones in skulls with artificial cranial deformation.

Near the posterior end of the sagittal suture are found two small openings called the parietal foramina. Normally these may be absent or faintly marked. Rarely they are greatly enlarged (Pancoast et al., 1940:9). These *enlarged parietal foramina* have been confused with bone disease and trephining. Another defect that may be mistaken for bone disease is *bilateral thinning of the parietals*. This is described by Thomas Lodge (Brothwell and Sandison 1967:chap. 31) and by Don Brothwell (Brothwell and Sandison 1967:Chap. 32). The areas of thinning can be of various sizes, are usually roughly circular in shape, are bilateral but not necessarily symmetrical, and will appear as shallow cup-like depressions. *Multiple infraorbital, ethmoidal* (anterior and posterior), and *mental foramina* are very common anomalies. According to Riesenfeld (1956) the percentage of multiple foramina in man varies in different populations from 6 to 33.12.

The vertebrae are the site of frequent and various congenital defects. These are more numerous in the cervical and lumbar areas. Most are considered to be the result of a development error in one or more of the many ossification centers in a growing vertebra.

A fusion of the *atlas* to the *occipital bone* is a rare occurrence (Plate 5,C). In life, if the fusion is complete, there is usually no disability (Epstein 1962, Chap. 2).

Occasionally there may be fusion or a lack of segmentation of other segments of the cervical vertebrae. (See Epstein 1962 and Pancoast 1940.) A severe manifestation of this deformity is called the *Klippel-Feil* syndrome which clinically may be characterized by shortness of the neck, limitation in movement, pain and generalized neurologic disturbances.

Many deviations from normal occur in cervical vertebrae. In reviewing some of the skeletal collection stored or on exhibit at Dickson Mounds, the following minor abnormalities were observed:

(1) Absence of one or more tubercles
(2) Incomplete transverse foramen
(3) Double transverse foramen
(4) Lack of segmentation of two vertebrae
(5) Failure of fusion of the posterior neural arch of the atlas
(6) Partial or complete enclosure by bone to change the groove for the vertebral artery to a foramen
(7) Fusion or lack of segmentation of the spine of two adjoining vertebrae
(8) Deformity of the dens
(9) Malposition of the odontoid facet

The most frequently encountered abnormalities in the lumbosacral area are: partial or complete fusion of the fifth lumbar to the sacrum; a diminution or increase in the number of sacral segments; and spina bifida. *Sacralization of the fifth lumbar* is characterized by apparently one additional sacral segment and one less lumbar vertebrae. The opposite is true in the condition called *lumbarization of the first sacral segment.*

Spina bifida is a defect in the posterior bony arch of the spine through which may protrude the meninges (meningocele) and neural structures (myelomeningocele). The presence of a meningocele or a myelomeningocele results in severe neurological symptoms and is incompatible with long life; so when an archaeologist finds such a defect in an adult skeleton, it can be safely assumed that the condition was a *spina bifida occulta* (Plate 23,B). A spina bifida occulta is characterized by a (usually small) defect in the posterior arch of the spine with no herniation and with no symptoms. This is common and is most frequently located in the upper segments of the sacrum and the fifth lumbar vertebra. According to Shands (1952:275), it is estimated that significant spina bifida occurs about once in every thousand births. Minor involvement of the upper sacral segment is found so often in archaeological specimens that these could be considered within the limits of normal.

In thoracic and lumbar vertebrae several rare congenital anomalies are found (Epstein 1962: Chap. 2). The most common is called *block vertebrae,* which is a fusion of two adjoining vertebrae to form one block. A *wedge vertebra* occurs when the anterior portion of the vertebral body fails to ossify properly, resulting in a triangle-shaped section of bone with the apex directed anteriorly. This creates a gibbus or angular deformity, which should be distinguished from tuberculosis since the bone edges would be smooth and there would be no evidence of bone destruction or regeneration. Two other conditions which would be difficult to differentiate from congenital wedging would be vertebral epiphysitis and vertebral osteochondritis. A *hemivertebra* is formed because of the failure of a vertebral body to ossify laterally. The resulting triangle has the apex pointing laterally to one side or the other. A *butterfly vertebra* (rare) follows defective ossification of the center. The appearance is of two triangles with apices directed inward, as in the wings of a butterfly.

Congenital rib abnormalities are quite common. The incidence, according to Table 4, is about 7 out of every 1,000 (Morse 1944). These include cervical, rudimentary, bifid, joined and broadened ribs. The data in Table

4 were taken from a careful analysis of 223,182 chest x-rays of Selective Service registrants taken at Camp Shelby, Mississippi, during World War II. Of these, 118,024 were white and 105,158 were nonwhite. It is interesting to note that of a total of 452 cervical ribs (about 2 out of every 1,000) only one had symptoms that could be interpreted as resulting from the rib defect. Truly congenital rib anomalies can be considered inconsequential.

Perforation of the coronoid-olecranon septum is encountered frequently in archaeological specimens (Plate 23,C). A racial or genetic occurrence is obvious. Glanville (1967) reports a 6 percent frequency of septal perforation in a group of European skeletons and a 47 percent incidence in skeletal material taken from some caves near Sanga in Mali (Africa). It would appear that individuals with less robust and more delicate bones have the higher incidence (Glanville 1967; and Benfer and McKern 1966). This condition is more frequent in females within the same population group. The antiquity of this defect is demonstrated in an article written by Dr. Holm Neumann (1967) describing the paleopathology of the inhabitants of the Modoc Rock Shelter. Although Dr. Neumann did not give the incidence of perforated septum in some 28 burials examined, two examples of humeri pictured in the photographic plates show the presence of large perforated foramina. One (Ra501-15) was female and the other (Ra501-20) was male. In a cursory preliminary analysis of late Archaic burials at the Morse Site, Fulton County, Illinois, the incidence of perforated olecranon foramina was high (28.6 percent). In some 28 burials complete enough to be included (11 males and 17 females), one male (9 percent) and 7 females (41 percent) had this congenital abnormality. The male skeletons at the Morse Site appear to have much larger bones with quite prominent ridges, crests and muscular impressions (*robust*) than do the bones of the females, which are small and delicate. Glanville further states that the presence of perforations are more frequent in those with a greater total angle of movement at the elbow from full extension to full flexion.

TABLE 4

SUMMARY OF CONGENITAL RIB ABNORMALITIES NOTED

	NUMBER		
	WHITE	NON-WHITE	TOTAL
Cervical ribs (Note: One is attached to the third cervical spine)	200	252	452
Rudimentary first ribs (Note: One is a rudimentary *third* rib)	117	54	171
Bifid ribs	257	328	585
Joined ribs	118	63	181
Broadened ribs	93	58	151
Miscellaneous congenital rib abnormalities	30	22	52
TOTAL	815	777	1592
PERCENT	.6905	.750	.7133

A developmental error in ossification is thought to be the cause of *perforation of the sternum*. This is encountered occasionally in archaeological material and appears as a smooth-bordered hole located in the body of the sternum.

Congenital *radio-ulnar synostosis* occurs when the proximal ends of the ulna and the radius are fused. Two examples of this defect are in the Dickson Mounds collection. Both are from the Crable Site and both involve the left arm (Fig. 4).

Two of the more disabling congenital deformities (Shands 1952: Chap. II) seen in archaeological specimens are *congenital dislocation of the hip* and *clubfoot*. Dislocation of the hip has been discussed in Chapter 2 under *trauma*. It would be difficult to tell always whether the dislocation was congenital or acquired. The one shown in Plate 6,B must have been of congenital origin, principally because it is bilateral. Bone changes due to dislocation can include: deformity and/or atrophy of the head of the femur; a shallowness of the acetabulum—sometimes filled with trabeculated bone whose appearance gives no

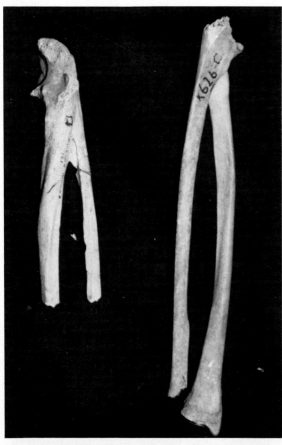

Fig. 4. Congenital radio-ulnar synostosis. (Both are left.) Crable Site, Fulton County, Illinois. Dickson Mounds Collection.

evidence of articulation; and a hollow depression on the anterior aspect of the ilium, forming a false socket for the displaced femoral head.

Congenital clubfoot is a gross deformity of the foot present at birth (Turek 1959). The most common type (up to 95 percent) is described as *talipes equinovarus* (the foot being plantar-flexed and inverted). *Talipes* means foot and ankle. *Equinus* is plantar flexion (toes pointed downward), and *varus* means inversion of the foot so that the bottom of the foot deviates medially. The other deformities are described by a combination of terms. *Calcaneus* is dorsal flexion of the foot (the toes pointing upward) and *valgus* is eversion of the foot. Thus the less common types are called: *talipes calcaneovalgus, talipes calcaneovarus* and *talipes equinovalgus.*

Deformities in the shape of individual bones of the feet will be apparent in a long-standing (neglected) talipes equinovarus. These variations in shape, which in themselves will vary greatly in the degree of severity, are dependent on: (1) the original genetic factor; (2) the adaptation of all bones of the foot and lower leg because of the original deformities; and (3) the adaptation of the bones of the foot and leg caused by usage.

Features of the clubfoot available to the clinician, such as shortening of ligaments and tendons and obvious abnormalities in foot position, are not available to the archaeologist. X-rays of the living foot may give false impressions of individual bone shapes, because the deformity causes the x-ray picture to be taken at an abnormal angle. Another difficulty in making an archaeological diagnosis is an apparent lack of availability of modern cases of untreated clubfeet. All have had manipulation therapy; this manipulation itself may cause bone-shape changes which otherwise would not occur.

In 1963, Irani and Sherman published a "classic" report, *The Pathological Anatomy of Club Foot.* Their findings were based on a dissection of 11 cases of clubfoot and 14 normal extremities. All were from stillbirths or neonatal deaths, ranging in menstrual age from 22 to 36 weeks. The only bone that was always abnormal was the *talus,* and it was suggested that this was the *"primary fault."* The most "conspicuous and constant abnormality" is that the neck of the talus is shortened and sometimes absent so that the head seems fused directly to the body; the angle which the long axis of the forepart of the talus makes with the long axis of the body is significantly decreased and the anterior portion of the talus is rotated in the medial and plantar direction. So-called secondary adaptive changes include: slight shape changes in the body of the talus; a shortening and widening of the calcaneous; and a decrease in the size of the navicular bone. Among other recorded changes are medial curving of the metatarsals, a flattening of the distal articular surface of the tibia, and a posterior displacement of the fibula.

In suspect cases the archaeologist should attempt to realign the foot and ankle bones, and compare them to the other foot or to a set of bones from a normal foot.

In a personal communication with Dr. Charles Snow, University of Kentucky, four cases of clubfoot and two instances of dislocated hip joints were found among some 1,200 pre-European Polynesian skeletons, principally from the sand dunes at Mokapu, Oahu, Hawaii (Collection of Bishop Museum, Honolulu). (See also Bowers 1966).

There is a group of abnormalities termed *bone dysplasias,* presumed to be caused by some developmental error in growing bone. It is assumed that most of these are inborn or genetic—although some may not be apparent at the time of birth. Different names have been assigned to the same defect by different authorities and many entities manifest various degrees of severity. Some of these variations have been given different names. Classification of these bone dysplasias have been attempted, one of the best being Rubin's *Modeling Sketches and Skeletons in the Dynamic Classification of Bone Dysplasias* (1964). It is probable that some of these "bone dysplasias" may be responsible for the occasional bizarre diagnosis-defying abnormalities encountered when one attempts to examine a large skeleton collection. Most of these "congenital errors of bone development" are extremely rare. Only a few are mentioned here.

Osteopetrosis (marble bones) is characterized by a marked increase in bone density. In normal modeling of bone there is always a balance between bone resorption and bone apposition. In osteopetrosis it is thought that bone apposition proceeds normally, but there is inadequate resorption of calcified cartilage and newly formed bone, resulting in an increase in minerals, weight, fragility and a narrowing or obliteration of marrow spaces. There are two forms recognized: the *malignant* and *benign* (Moseley 1963; Hinkle 1957). The malignant form is present at birth and even starts *in utero.* Clinically there is anemia, frequent fractures, deafness and cranial nerve disorders. Death usually occurs early. The benign form persists into or begins in adulthood. Sometimes there are no symptoms except perhaps bone fractures. Bone involvement in the benign form need not be so generalized.

Osteopoikilosis (spotted bones) is an abnormality of the skeleton where there are numerous islands of increased bone densities measuring 2 to 10 mm. in diameter and concentrated in the epiphyses and metaphyses near the epiphyseal lines. These dense areas are rare in the bone shafts and seldom involve the skull. In dried bone they could be apparent in cross section, in breaks and by x-ray. Clinically, there are no symptoms.

In *Engelmann's disease* there is a symmetrical enlargement of the shafts of the long bones with sclerosis. The error in modeling is an excess of periosteal bone formation. The long bones most frequently involved are the femora and the tibiae. Next common are the radiae, ulnae and fibulae. Hands, feet and spine usually escape involvement. The periosteum lays down new bone, causing an increase in the diameter and a decrease in the medullary spaces.

Infantile cortical hyperostosis (Caffey's disease) is a localized thickening of the periosteum and hyperplasia of underlying lamellar bone in young infants (Staheli et al 1968). It is self-limited and probably not inherited. The cause is unknown. The mandible is the most frequently involved bone. The bone changes are reversible, but occasionally they may persist, such as asymmetry of the lower jaw.

Osteogenosis imperfecta (brittle bones) is a failure of periosteal intramembranous bone formation (Rubin 1964). This disorder is characterized by an increase in bone fragility, resulting in multiple fractures frequently following the slightest trauma. There are numerous deformities caused by the fractures and callus formation. The disease is more severe in childhood. There is a thinning of the bone cortex and a widening of the medullary cavities. The bones appear normal in length, but the diameter of the long bones is diminished.

The author knows of no cases of osteogenesis imperfecta occurring in the Midwest; but Brothwell suggests a possibility in an Egyptian case (Brothwell and Sandison 1967:Chap. 34, p. 441), and Wells (Brothwell and Sandison 1967:Chap. 43, p. 525) diagnosed an osteogenesis imperfecta from an Anglo-Saxon cemetery.

Achondroplasia is caused by a failure of proliferative cartilage (Rubin 1964). This is the well-recognized form of dwarfism with a shortening of the long tubular bones and with an apparently normal-sized head and trunk. Since periosteal bone formation is unaffected, the diameter of the long bones appears normal, creating the illusion of thick diaphyses. Since only the base of the skull is cartilaginous in its development (Pugh 1958), there is a delayed growth in this area. The face may be disproportionately small with prognathism (projecting jaw) (Rubin 1964). The etiology is unknown, but there is a definite hereditary factor (Luck 1950). Clinically, the dwarf has a normal intelligence with a congenial nature. He has an abbreviated stature, large head, pug nose and stubby fingers, arms and legs. When a normal person stands upright with his hands at his sides, the tips of his fiñers reach to about mid-thigh. The arms of of the achondroplastic dwarf are so short that his fingers will reach to about the level of the iliac crests. This type of dwarf was well known in ancient times in both the Old and the New World. Two prehistoric American Indian achondroplastic dwarf skeletons, one male and one female, were reported in detail by Charles E. Snow (1943) from the University of Kentucky. They were excavated from the Moundsville Site, Alabama, and belonged to the Mississippian Culture.

Miscellaneous Defects

Spondylolysis is a defect in the interarticular portion of the neural arch. (See Plate 22,C and D.) This occurs almost always in the fifth lumbar vertebra, but in rare cases will occur in the other lumbar vertebrae. The condition is almost always bilateral, that is, occurring on both sides of the neural arch, although very rarely there may be a unilateral break. Apparently spondylolysis in itself gives no symptoms. The separated arch can be held in place by surrounding tissues and ligaments. When there is a displacement forward or backward of the upper vertebra in relationship to the lower segment (in case of the fifth lumbar the lower segment would be the sacrum), symptoms may develop. The condition is now called *spondylolisthesis* (derived from the Greek: *spondylus,* vertebra; and *olisthesis,*

slipping). The symptoms can be mild or severe and can include pain, stiffness of the back and a waddling gait.

The etiology of spondylolysis has never been definitely determined, but most authorities believe that there is some contributing genetic factor (Wiltse 1957; Stewart 1956; Epstein 1962; Ritvo 1955; Merbs and Wilson 1960; Rowe and Roche 1953). This abnormality does not exist at birth. Rowe and Roche (1953) report no defective arches in over 500 infant cadavers. In addition, there is no ossification center located in the arch where the break occurs. Fractures do occur in the neural arch due to trauma, but not in the same location as the separation in spondylolysis. In addition, there is a definite familial (Wiltse 1957) and racial variation. Rowe and Roche (1953) report an overall 5 percent incidence of spondylolysis in the study of 4,200 skeletons. The white males had the highest incidence, 6.4 percent, and Negro females the lowest, 1.1 percent. Stewart (1956) reports an extraordinarily high incidence of neural arch defects in skeletons of Alaskan natives ranging from 15 to 50 percent, according to geographic area. Lester and Shapiro (1968) report an incidence of 21 percent in the prehistoric Ipiutak Eskimos and 45 percent in the Tigara who existed about 1,000 years later. Snow (1948) reports 17 percent of separate neural arch in males and 20 percent in females in the Indian Knoll skeletons. In the Morse Red Ocher Site (Mound 772), there were 5 spondylolyses of the 16 skeletons complete enough to be counted, or 31 percent. It should be noted that this figure at the Morse Site is only tentative because of the small number of skeletons and the extreme disturbance by rodents.

Extra facets or *pseudarthroses* can be classified as pathological or physiological. Pathological facets can occur whenever there is a derangement of a joint or bone through some developmental error or trauma such as fracture or dislocation, so that two surfaces abnormally appose each other. All extra facets could actually be called physiological as there is an attempt on the part of the body to compensate for some abnormal influence. The best and almost the only examples of physiological facets are those brought about by "squatting."

In a long-standing dislocation of the hip, either congenital or acquired (Plate 6,A and B), a false acetabulum can form on the surface of the ilium to accommodate the displaced head of the femur. In a shoulder dislocation or an acromioclavicular separation, a formation of extra facets may result. (See Plate 6,G.) A good example of a pseudarthrosis following a fracture is illustrated in Plate 4,(3). Here the fracture of the right ulna did not heal properly and a new joint resulted, supplying a rigid support to the fracture, resulting in very little actual disability.

In the excavation at Dickson Mounds during the summer of 1966, a male, age 50 (F34-309) had a congenital failure of fusion of the posterior arch of the atlas. Apparently this caused a lateral displacement, which resulted in the formation of a pseudo-joint between the right side of the dens and the adjacent portion of the atlas. Plate 23,A shows the presence of a facet on the anterior lower end of the tibia, apparently due to a deformity of the foot and a shortening of the right tibia. This facet is in the same location found in so-called *squatting facets;* however, in this instance, it is caused by the foot deformity.

In some primitive and ancient cultures the habit of squatting with the feet flat on the ground and the buttocks resting on the heels results in the formation of squatting facets due to a long-existing, over-extension of joints bringing surfaces in apposition. These facets usually occur in three locations (Fig. 5). The most common is the anterior distal end of the tibia and a connecting facet in the talus. The other locations are at the knee, usually on the medial side of the proximal end of the tibia, with a companion facet on the distal end of the femur; and a small area of depression on the anterior medial surface of the head of the femur, at about the junction of the head and neck, with a companion facet on the anterior medial portion of the acetabulum. There may be another facet on the posterior head of the femur. These facets at the hip are called "Poirier's facets." Snow (1948) reports that 95 percent of the adult Indian Knolls skeletons had squatting facets at the ankle, and Poirier's facets occurred in 59.4 percent of the males and 40.7 percent of the females. Harris, in 1948, found nearly 50 percent occurrence

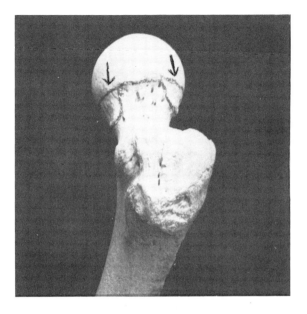

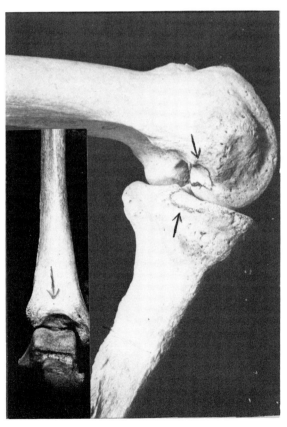

Fig. 5. Squatting facets. Hip, knee and ankle (anterior view). *Photograph, courtesy Dr. Charles Snow.*

of squatting facets among the Huron Indians. Not many skeletal collections in the Midwest show the presence of squatting facets, but King Hunter found them to be rather frequent among the Klunk Site prehistoric Indians.

Artificial cranial deformities can be accidental, i.e., caused by the weight of the infant's head against the cradleboard, or by intentional means, such as headbinding. Almost any form and degree of deformity can occur artificially (Fig. 6). The shapes most often encountered are as follows (Snow 1941; Neumann 1942):

Occipital. The occipital bone is flattened because the infant's head lies against the cradleboard. The flattening can be centered (symmetrical) or off-center (asymmetrical), depending on the position assumed by the child's head against the board.

Bifronto-occipital. The occipital bone is flat and there is a flattened area on both sides of the frontal bone caused by the back of the head lying against a cradleboard and two other boards bound one to each side of the forehead, resulting in a triangle-shaped skull when viewed from above.

Fronto-vertico-occipital. This is brought about by intentional binding on a cradleboard, with or without the use of an additional board placed in the frontal area. (See Plate 23,D.)

Parallelo-fronto-occipital. This is supposed to result from placing a "pad" at the base of the occiput to cause the flattened occipital bone to slope backward, and probably another board is bound to the forehead so that the flattened area of the frontal is roughly parallel to the plane of the occipital deformation. This usually results in a broadened skull.

Lambdoidal. This deformation is characterized by a flattened lambdoidal region as opposed to the straight occipital, a variation of cradleboard deformity (Stewart 1940). (See Plate 23,E.)

Fronto-parieto-occipital. The occipital flattening is caused by the cradleboard; the other flat areas are the result of a board being placed on top of the skull and another in front. Lateral compensatory growth will take place (Stewart 1941:93).

Variously shaped intentional deformations. These could conceivably be the result of binding with eccentrically placed boards or—as in Snow's pre-Captain Cook Hawaiians—binding with cut coconut shells (Bowers 1966).

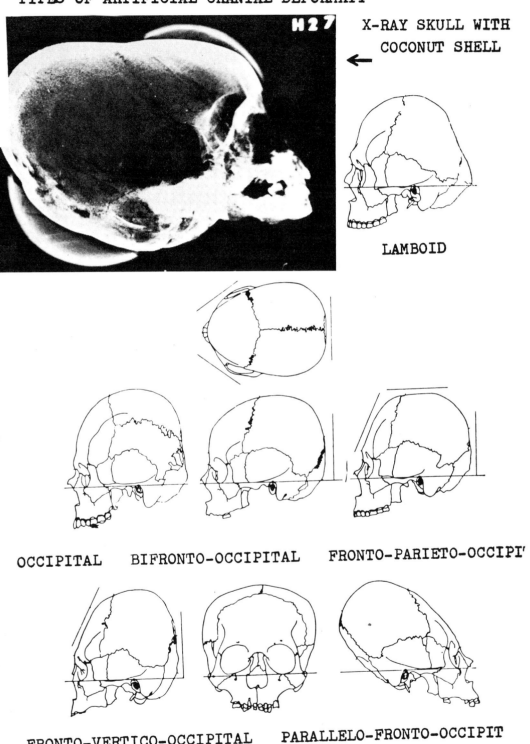

X-RAY SKULL WITH
COCONUT SHELL

LAMBOID

OCCIPITAL   BIFRONTO-OCCIPITAL   FRONTO-PARIETO-OCCIPI'

FRONTO-VERTICO-OCCIPITAL   PARALLELO-FRONTO-OCCIPIT

Fig. 6. Artificial cranial deformations. *X-ray, courtesy Dr. Charles Snow.*

CHAPTER 8

DENTAL PATHOLOGY OF THE EARLY INDIAN POPULATIONS OF THE MIDWEST

Albert A. Dahlberg, D.D.S.*

It can be concluded from the conditions seen on the teeth of the early Midwest Indians that their diet was basically good and that there was no severe debilitating disease during the period of development in childhood. This speaks well for their environment and the understanding they must have had of body nutritional needs. However, in every group of living beings there are to be found some who are less sturdy and less resistant to impacts of disease and their surroundings. Among the large number of well-documented teeth and skulls of the Dickson Mounds collection, there are many examples of pathology of significance and interest.

Many of the pathological conditions discussed in the previous chapters apply to teeth as well as to bone. The differences of structure, composition, use and the relationships of other tissues, of course, are very apparent. Additionally, teeth are frequently used as tools and are subjected to environmental contacts much contrasted to the soft, tissue-covered bone.

In approaching the problem of paleopathological studies of the dentition, one does not have all the tools of the modern clinician such as the many sophisticated bacteriologic, histologic and chemical tests. With the increase in knowledge and refinement of technical procedures, some of these difficulties are being overcome. This is seen in the chemical analyses of bone constituents and blood residues that are now possible. However, for the most part, available approaches are confined to visual, microscopic and x-ray techniques.

From the literature we have obtained a perspective of the incidences of the more obvious dental pathologies in the Paleolithic, Neolithic and Recent periods. Some of the conditions found are rare and occur only in certain areas. Classifying them is helpful to understanding.

Paleopathology of the dentition can be categorized in nine general groups:

(1) Conditions imposed on the dentition and surrounding tissues by bacteria and their by-products.

(2) Invasion of tissues by overgrowth of a tissue (neoplasm).

(3) Conditions induced by extraneous objects or substances (calcular accumulations).

(4) Atrophy of tissues (aging, disuse).

(5) Normal or excessive wear and use.

(6) Results of mechanical alteration or violence (extractions, fractures, decorations).

(7) Developmental phenomena (nutrition, trace elements, accidents in development, incidental abberation and other factors affecting the units during development).

(8) Genetic characterizations (agenesis).

(9) Other conditions (tori, exostoses, etc.).

These nine categories will be considered in a little more detail.

Conditions Imposed by Bacteria and Their By-products

Although the dental caries rate was not excessively high, *decay* and *abscesses* did occur. The conditions imposed on the dentition and surrounding tissues by bacteria and their by-products are in evidence in the early Midwest Indians. In the proper environment of heat, moisture and carbohydrates decay in a tooth generally progresses through the pain-responding dentin and pulp tissues to the areas around the root ends. Here the bacterial invasion is met by combating blood and tissue elements in an attempt to isolate the process. The infection, depending on the virulence of the organism, may under the physical pressure

*Acting Director, Zoller Memorial Dental Clinic and Research Associate (Professor), Department of Anthropology, University of Chicago.

created within the tissues by its own by-products and bacterial multiplication, force a path through the bone and soft tissues to the outside with the resultant purulent discharge. The result of this process seen in skeletal material is a cavity in the bone in the vicinity of the root ends (Plate 26,F). Bacteria of lesser virulence can be less violent with an even, well-circumscribed small area around the apices in contrast to the other larger bone cavities. Infections can also gain entrance to the tissues around the teeth by way of the gums, particularly where health-sustaining vitamins might have been lacking in the diets or where the gums might have been penetrated by fragments in the masticating process. This sort of bacterial invasion rarely produces a cavity in the bone but rather causes recession of the supporting bone found between the teeth (Plate 25,F).

Invasion of Tissues by Overgrowth of a Tissue (Neoplasm)

Cavities of this type may be differentiated from the bacteria-produced ones by the character of their periphery and by the lack of association with a likely involved broken-down tooth. X-ray can be useful in such diagnoses. The extent of the process will sometimes indicate the nature of the neoplasm such as the compartmentalized interlocular cyst. Extensive involvement of cavities with obvious destruction of bone in adjacent areas is apt to be indicative of malignant processes. One can not always distinguish the chronic-suppurative from the neoplastic lesions.

Conditions Induced by Extraneous Objects or Substances

Deposits of calcified salts are frequently found around the gum margins of teeth (Plate 27,A). This is commonly known as "tartar" and "calculus." It irritates the gum tissues, causing them to become inflamed. This in turn causes the bony support between the teeth to resorb, the topmost part becoming flat. The process continues until after varying periods of time the support is weakened and the teeth become loose and drift into other positions, generally anteriorly. The ultimate result is loss of the tooth or teeth.

Impactions of pieces of foreign materials such as wood or even food between the teeth will also cause recession of bone. Not only is resorption observed in the presence of inflammatory conditions but also activity of bone-building cells is induced on a minor scale. Small islands of exostoses (Plate 27,A) may be observed along the bony edges of teeth and in areas subjected to traumatic impacts.

Teeth may be moved apart in their alignment when a tissue growth (benign or malignant) grows between them. This is not infrequent in the case of epuli, which are benign fibrous-tissue growths. Teeth of the opposing arch sometimes cause tooth movement or spread also. The spacing between the upper central incisors of Plate 25,A is similar to such a condition as is sometimes found with epuli, although in this instance it probably is associated with whatever this individual did to produce the worn notches on the incisal edges of the upper and lower left incisor teeth.

Atrophy of Tissues

Bones, particularly the alveolar processes, atrophy markedly in the circumstances of aging. Atrophy also occurs as a result of overuse, disuse and as a symptom of certain internal gland problems such as uncontrolled diabetes. The teeth in such cases are found to be in good condition but lacking support because of the diffuse atrophy of the alveolus throughout the dentition. Plate 26, E and G, illustrate the atrophy of the ridges from disuse. The x-ray (G) reveals a root fragment which rules out the possibility posed formerly that this person never had any teeth.

Normal or Excessive Wear and Use

In many areas and populations of the past, wear of the teeth and attrition of the supporting tissues proceeded much more rapidly than they do today. In some skeletal materials it is obvious, from the wear pattern, that the function of mastication was confined to one area for a length of time and subsequently shifted to another as each locale in sequence succumbed to the heavy demands and wear by abscessing or otherwise breaking down. The lower jaws of Plate 25,E, and Plate 27,D, show this clearly.

Teeth wear mainly in two places: the occlusal surface, where the masticating takes place (Plate 27,F) and at the points of contact between each tooth and its neighbor. As the supporting structure weakens, the teeth shift in position as mentioned previously.

Results of Mechanical Alteration or Violence

Decoration (notching on Plate 25,B) was not as common in the Midwest as in other parts of Early America. Accidental or deliberate removal of teeth allows the opposing and adjacent teeth to shift toward the vacancy. This invites caries and interdental pocket formation from food accumulations between the teeth. Efficiency of the occlusal function is decreased as the teeth tip away at angles. A whole array of changes take place in the region and ultimately, in many cases, leads to infection. A very unusual result of deliberate removal of teeth is seen in some groups of people such as the Afalou in Africa, all of whom had their upper incisor teeth removed. The Midwest Indians never did this. In the Afalou this allowed for an overeruption and higher position of the unopposed lower teeth whose incisal edges also took on a peculiarly slanted angle of wear as a result of the lateral movements with new tooth relationships. In movement of teeth the supporting alveolar bone follows and changes with the new tooth position. This is evident in the Afalou, in whom the anterior part of the mandible in the incisor region elongated in the already large structure to give a reversed rodent appearance. Loss of teeth in other parts of the jaw give the same effect, i.e., overeruption of the unopposed ones. Sites of fracture can usually be detected and are frequently indicative of the nature of the blow which produced them. One of the well-known instances was in the Australopithecines, in which the fractures in the lower right and left premolar regions gave all the earmarks of a hard blow on the anterior part of the jaw. A blow from the side will frequently produce a fracture of the neck of the condyle of the opposite side.

Developmental Phenomena

These include such conditions found in the teeth and supporting bone which are due to interruptions, disturbances, nutritional deficiencies, hormonal imbalances, or other circumstances occurring during the development of the tissues. A dentigerous (follicular) cyst is typical of this and involves the formation of a cystic cavity associated with the crown of the tooth rather than the root, as in bacteria-induced cavities. Other developmental phenomena include such things as cleft palates, deformities of the jaws, impacted or misplaced teeth (Plate 26,C and D, and Plate 27,F), deformation of roots, hypoplastic teeth, mottled enamel and many asymmetries of bone and tooth form. Figures C and D show a most unusual malposition. In none of the specimens at Dickson Mounds was there any evidence of mottling from fluoride.

Clefts in palates range from small openings to complete separation of the two sides. Occasionally, an incomplete closure of the premaxillae is observed so that the alveolar bone of the two maxillary incisors are semi-independent of each other and give an appearance of a terminal situation of each of the right and left halves of the dentition. Microscopic details of teeth are influenced by nutritional and other variables during development also.

An enamel pearl (development from remnant enamel-forming cells) is seen on the mesial surface of Plate 25,D. In addition to the numerical variation of congenital absence of teeth, there are instances of increased number—supernumerary teeth. These are illustrated in Plate 26,H and Plate 25,C.

Genetic Characterizations

Genetically based variations of the teeth and jaws are frequently found and include alterations in number, size and form. Plate 26,H shows an extra upper lateral incisor in jaws that are too small for the size of the teeth. This results in the crowding and irregularities in the position of the teeth. The most commonly missing teeth are the upper lateral incisors, the third molars and the second premolars. A long list of other genetic characteristics includes the cusps, roots and pulp chambers such as the taurodont characteristic. Taurodontism (large root and pulp chamber) was not observed in the Indians. The large ridges in the cupped-out inner (lingual) surfaces of the upper incisors are seen in Plate 26,H.

These are termed "shovel shaped." (See also Plate 27, D,E.)

A foremost characteristic of the teeth of Indians is the shape of the incisor previously mentioned. Plate 27,D shows an additional feature, the barrel-shaped lateral incisor (upper right). This form is sometimes huge, frequently resembling a premolar in size and form. Another feature seen with high frequency in Indian dentitions is an extra cusp or modification of it on the anterior cheek side (mesial of the buccal) of the buccal surfaces of the lower molars. These and other characteristics occur in a pattern of greater to lesser degree of size and expression from the first to the third molars. Carabelli's cusps in the Dickson Mounds collection were small to absent.

Other Conditions

Another group of conditions related to the dentition include certain *exostoses* which are not classed as neoplasms or as developmental phenomena. These are the *tori* of the midline of the maxilla, those of the lingual aspect of the alveolar bone of the mandible, and a third group of lesser incidence which occurs on the buccal surfaces of the alveolar ridges. The maxillary tori are sometimes confused with irregularity and prominence of the median raphe, the suture line between the palatal processes of the right and left maxillae. The mandibular tori always occur above the mylohyoid ridge and in greatest evidence in the canine and premolar areas. The buccal exostoses are limited to the vicinity of the premolars and molars (Plate 27,A). These structures on skeletal material are difficult to compare to those in the living because of the masking effect of the overlaid soft tissues. They range from small, simple nodes to large pedunculated masses up to 4 by 6 cm. in size. There are also small irregularities of bone in the palate, of no apparent significance but present nevertheless. These are not present in the early midwestern peoples. Acromegaly is a condition involving the disproportionate enlarging of the mandible and other bones in adults.

Excessive pounding (traumatic occlusion) of a tooth by its opponent can also be responsible for bony changes, especially on the thin labial and buccal bony plates.

The temporomandibular joint is a structure closely related to the dentition. Pathology of the craniomandibular articulation is often associated with dental alterations. Pathologic change, involving the bony parts of the articulation, may be observed in the condylar process of the mandible and on the squamous and zygomatic portions of the temporal bone. Among the pathologic conditions which affect the bony elements of the temporomandibular articulation are fractures of the condyle, which disturb the growth and development of the mandible. Bony ankylosis of the mandibular joint may result from such traumatic experiences.

Other pathologies that existed in life, particularly in soft tissues, leave little or no evidence. Muscle attachments offer clues to muscular involvements. Overuse of one side of the dentition is frequently an indication of an atrophic oropathologic condition of the opposite side. The effect of overfunction on the "used" side is readily observed.

A systematic approach to dental paleopathology can assist in differentiating paleopopulations and perhaps can be useful in the understanding of some related pathological conditions. Dental paleopathology is helpful in evaluating environmental influences and habits which affect the dentition.

The assemblage of dentitions in the ancient Midwest ranged from the most beautiful, well-aligned and well-proportioned set in Plate 26,A, to the very extreme crowding and disproportion shown in Plate 26,H. Most of the dentitions were well aligned and very functional, with a relatively small incidence of dental caries. Periodontal disease was present in varying degree and measure—some extreme, especially in the older individuals. Abscesses and tooth loss were common in the elderly. Wear was extreme and typical of a diet having a high abrasive content.

Chapter 9

SPECIFIC DISEASES

This chapter will discuss principally two diseases: *tuberculosis* and *treponema infection*. By treponema infection we include yaws and syphilis because, as far as bone pathology is concerned, these two cannot be satisfactorily separated from one another. It has been demonstrated in early literature, in art forms, and in actual pathological specimens, that tuberculosis existed for thousands of years in the Old World; however, there is no completely convincing evidence that the disease was present in the Americas before the time of Columbus. The origin of syphilis is more controversial. It would appear, from the accumulation of excavated pathological specimens, that some sort of treponema infection probably did exist in the pre-Columbian New World.

Tuberculosis

Dr. J. Vernon Luck (1950), in *Bone and Joint Diseases,* makes the following statement: "The clinical diagnosis of skeletal tuberculosis is not a simple matter, and according to published statistics, a substantial percentage of error occurs even in the best of our orthopedic clinics."

If one is confronted solely with a dried bone specimen, this error will certainly be multiplied many times. Furthermore, if one attempted to make a diagnosis from a prehistoric bone specimen, the only chance of making even a good guess would be if there were involvement of the spine. Tuberculosis in other locations would be indistinguishable from too many other diseases. It is true that tuberculosis involving the spine can cause different pathological results, depending on virulence of the organism and resistance of the victim. If the host had little ability to defend himself, then tuberculosis could cause a rapidly progressive type of acute osteomyelitis, re-

sulting in early death. If the host's resistance was considerable, it is presumed that the disease then would be extra-chronic, with the possibility of extensive healing and bone regeneration. Between these two extremes lies the pathologic picture of what is said to be typical spinal tuberculosis, without which it is impossible to make even a presumptive diagnosis of tuberculosis in a dried bone specimen.

Some characteristics of spinal tuberculosis:

(1) Tuberculosis of the spine usually involves one to four vertebrae. Involvement of more vertebrae does occur, but this is rare.

(2) Bone destruction occurs with little or no bone regeneration.

(3) As the disease advances, the bone in the vertebral bodies becomes eroded and decalcified. Under the pressure of body weight the spine collapses forward, giving the characteristic deformity, the angular kyphosis (Figure 7).

(4) Involvement of the neural arches and transverse and spinous processes is rare.

(5) Extravertebral "cold" abscesses are frequent. In the cervical and upper dorsal region these can occur posteriorly, and the sinus tracts can open externally. In the lower thoracic and lumbar areas, abscesses will develop anteriorly and occasionally rupture into the peritoneal cavity or proceed to the psoas area, but they will almost never open through the skin posteriorly.

(6) Massive regeneration of the bone is a great rarity, and even spontaneous fusion is uncommon. That is why, before tuberculosis of the bone was treated with specific antituberculous drugs, so many cases necessitated surgical intervention.

Many other conditions can be confused with spinal tuberculosis, especially if only the dried bone specimens are available. Among the diseases that would have to be considered in a differential diagnosis are:

Chronic pyogenic osteomyelitis
Traumatic arthritis
Crush fractures
Malignancy
Typhoid spine
Sarcoidosis
Actinomycosis
Blastomycosis
Coccidioidomycosis
Rheumatoid arthritis
Osteitis deformans (Paget's disease)
Osteochondritis
Neuroarthropathies

Kyphosis. In the past there was a widespread misconception that kyphosis was synonymous with spinal tuberculosis. The frequent references in literature that prehistoric hunchback art invariably means tuberculosis are not consistent with clinical facts. Besides the various diseases mentioned in the differential diagnosis table, developmental, nutritional, and endocrine disturbances are more frequent causes of all sorts of spinal deformities, including kyphosis, than is tuberculosis.

In Lincoln State School (an institution for the mentally retarded located in Lincoln, Illinois) there are many severe deformities of the spine among the residents. Four of the most severe kyphotic cases, which could resemble the models of prehistoric hunchback art, were selected and are pictured in Plate 28. Roentgenographic interpretation was made by Dr. Edward Wood, consulting radiologist at Lincoln State School. None of the roentgenograms gave the remotest indication that tuberculosis was the cause of the deformity.

Expected frequency. Assuming that tuberculosis did exist in a prehistoric American population and also assuming that treatment was either absent or at a very low minimum, what can be expected as to the incidence of bone tuberculosis in the skeletal material excavated? Some statistics are available on the tuberculosis morbidity and mortality of Indians in the United States during the early 1900's. At this time, treatment for tubercu-

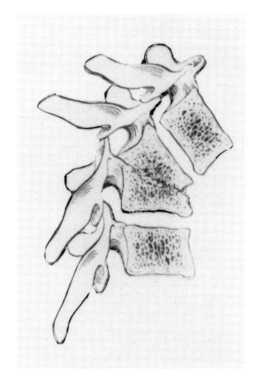

Fig. 7. Tuberculosis of the spine. Destruction of vertebral bodies resulting in the characteristic angular deformity. (Girdlestone 1940)

losis among Indians was practically nonexistent, and most of the Indians lived in close contact with one another in overcrowded homes scattered throughout reservations. These conditions would be somewhat similar to concentrations of Indian populations in some parts of prehistoric America, such as our South Central states, certain South American areas, and in the Southwest among the prehistoric Pueblo. The first statistics on this subject were presented by Dr. Ales Hrdlicka (1909), who collected 91 separate reports from physicians in the Indian Service during the years 1904 and 1908, involving an Indian population of 107,000.

Indian population 107,000
Pulmonary tuberculosis 1,038
Lymph-node tuberculosis 1,590
Bone tuberculosis   208

This report shows that 7 of every 100 cases of tuberculosis involved the bone and that there were 20 bone cases to every 100 pulmonary cases.

Valentine (1912) recorded that, of a total population of 183,587 Indians, there was a total of 5,960 deaths from all causes, and 1,905 deaths from tuberculosis. At that time, one of every three deaths among the Indians in the United States was caused by tuberculosis (rate 31.96). This would mean that in excavation of skeletal material, we could expect that, of every 1,000 deaths 320 would be caused by tuberculosis. According to Hrdlicka, 7 percent of all tuberculosis in living Indians involved the bone. This would suggest that 22.4 of every 1,000 burial specimens will show evidence of bone tuberculosis. Tuberculosis of the spine is the most frequent site of tuberculosis of the bone (more than 30 percent); thus, of every 1,000 excavated skeletons there should be about 6.7 cases of tuberculosis of the spine. These statistics, of course, are not foolproof. Obviously, in 1904 and 1908 there must have been many cases of missed diagnoses, and the misses as far as pulmonary disease is concerned would probably be greater than those of bone tuberculosis. In addition, we are comparing Hrdlicka's incidence of 1907-1908 with the mortality figures in the *Report of the Commissioner of Indian Affairs* (Valentine 1912). Another factor that might alter this presumption would be that it is not known how much tuberculosis in the Indians of 1912 was caused by the human or by the bovine tubercle bacilli, as the incidence of bone involvement is thought by some to be the highest when bovine bacilli are the cause. Regardless of the type of bacilli, bone involvement as a complication of pulmonary disease would be expected to be more prevalent when most of the cases were severe, advanced, and progressive.

Allowing for these statistical deficiencies, if prehistoric tuberculosis did exist in America, there should be many cases of typical spinal tuberculosis found among the large amount of excavated material.

Art Forms in America. Dr. Gerald B. Webb (1936), in his history of tuberculosis, makes the following statement which has been repeated frequently in the literature: "In pre-Columbian bronzes from Peru, in effigy water bottles in Indian burial grounds in many of our states, and from the pictographs of the cliff-dwellers, all pre-Columbian, the unmis-

takable picture of Potts' disease is portrayed. This picture is so characteristic that orthopedic surgeons are certain that tuberculosis alone can be the cause."

Pre-Columbian bronzes from Peru. The Inca of ancient Peru manufactured many metal and ceramic effigies and figurines depicting various diseases and deformities. The exact number of authentic hunchbacked figures from this area is unknown, but it is certain that they are very rare. Two are located in the U. S. National Museum. The figure of the man on the llama is 4½ inches tall and is made of silver. It came from Cuzco, Peru, and is pre-Spanish in time (Plate 28,H). The culture is Inca. Dr. Webb states that several of these bronzes are in the possession of the Army Medical Museum. One is illustrated in his book. However, after correspondence with the Curator of the Museum and a personal visit, only one bronze figure was found to be on exhibit, and no information as to its authenticity could be obtained. The figure pictured in Webb's book could not be located.

Hunchback art can be found sparsely scattered throughout Mexico and Central and South America. Instances of figurines, vases, and pottery vessels depicting spinal deformities have been located in Venezuela, Guatemala, and Costa Rica. Many of these may be historic. On some, it is doubtful that the intention was to portray deformity but may represent a natural position of bending over, or the desire on the part of the artist to create symmetry. Others strongly suggest a pack on the back and not a deformed spine.

Effigy water bottles (Plate 28). In a small area of central United States, including the corners of Arkansas, Tennessee, Mississippi, and Missouri, dozens of pottery bottles representing severely deformed hunchbacked human beings have been found by archaeologists. These water bottles have been identified as having been manufactured by people of a prehistoric Indian culture (Late Mississippian). However, some recent dating strongly suggests that at least some of these may have been post-Columbian in time. The Banks Site, Crittenden County, Arkansas, where many of these vessels were found, gave a carbon date of A.D. 1535. Artifacts found elsewhere in this "Memphis" area suggest that other sites may also have a late date. It might be assumed that the original potters used human beings as their models for these vessels. The literature contains many references that these hunchback bottles are evidence of the existence of tuberculosis in the American Indian before contact with the white man. The writer has personally seen many of these bottles and viewed photographs of many others. The majority do not show the typical angular deformity of tuberculosis but have smooth, rounded curves with the prominent individual spines evenly spaced throughout the curvatures,

Pictographs in the Southwest. In Plate 28 a pictograph group is shown which was found near Ruin 5 in Canyon Hagoe. Webb quoted these as representing spinal deformities due to tuberculosis with involvement of the cerebrospinal cord. Some of the group are pictured lying down, which is supposed to portray paralysis of the legs, and the playing on the flute is suggestive of occupational therapy. The figures which show priapism are supposed to be the result of spinal irritation. On the pictographs throughout the Southwest there have been many instances showing these hunchbacked flute players. From a medical standpoint, it is not likely that individuals with tuberculosis of the spine, in such an advanced stage as suggested in the pictures, would care much about lying on their backs playing flutes.

Elsie Parsons, in writing for *The American Anthropologist*, 1938, states that the hunchbacked flute player displayed on the rock walls throughout the Southwest is not a human being but represents an insect. This is the antecedent of the historic Hopi Katchina character called Kokopolo. The function of male Kokopolo is to chase women. Once he has seduced them he gives them a few presents, which he carries in his hump. According to Dr. Frank Roberts (1932) in a study of the historic Zuni, it is believed that the hunchbacked flute player may represent a rain priest, and that the frequently associated figures of horned toads and insects are symbols of magic. Furthermore, it is very likely that all of the pictographs in the Southwest made by prehistoric Indians were not meant to be accurate reproductions of certain objects but have a legendary or mythological meaning.

Skeletal Remains in Prehistoric America. The following fifteen cases of reported spinal tuberculosis in America are reviewed. Other cases undoubtedly are in existence, but their scarcity emphasizes the probability that tuberculosis was not the cause. Six of these cases could be considered as being found in the Midwest.

Case 1 (Putnam and Whitney). The first suggestion of tuberculosis in a prehistoric American Indian was from a published report by Dr. William F. Whitney of Harvard Medical School in 1886. Apparently, the Curator of the Peabody Museum, Dr. F. W. Putnam, asked Dr. Whitney to make a study of their osteologic collection. One skeleton, Cat. No. 17223, from a stone grave mound near Nashville, Tennessee, showed an extreme case of anterior angular spinal curvature. "The disease had destroyed almost the whole of the bodies of the lower cervical and upper dorsal vertebrae and they had then become united in a firm mass."

Two other specimens, both from Tennessee stone graves, were reported by Dr. Whitney. One involved the knee joint and the other the ankle. He concluded that these two were very suggestive of bone tuberculosis, but his description of the specimens did not justify this conclusion.

Case 2 (Plate 29,A) (Moore and Hrdlicka). Skeleton 277,730 is now located at the Department of Physical Anthropology, Smithsonian Institution, Washington, D. C. It was found by Clarence Moore in 1913 in a mound at Sorrel Bayou, Iberville Parish, Louisiana. The specimen was first examined and reported in 1913 by Ales Hrdlicka who described it as follows: "The bones of skeleton 277,730 show considerable disease. They represent what is either tuberculosis or a very pronounced form of arthritis at the lower dorsal and especially the upper lumbar vertebrae, with moderate curvature forward of the spine." In addition, Dr. Hrdlicka reports "an abscess cavity in the distal end of the left clavicle, more or less marked traces of periostitis of all the long bones, and signs of arthritis on one of the condyles of the right femur and lower articular surface at the right humerus." The bones represent one of the two skeletons in the mound which may belong to intrusive or later burials.

This specimen was seen and photographed by the author. All of the available vertebrae showed a moderate amount of osteoporosis and there was lipping of all bodies. Lumbar vertebrae Nos. 1, 2, 3, and 4 had a moth-eaten appearance on the surfaces of the bodies, with numerous tiny bony nodulations (see photograph). The pathologic appearance of this specimen has no resemblance to tuberculosis (Plate 29).

Case 3 (Hooton). This case was reported by Dr. Earnest Albert Hooton in 1930, and the specimen was from the large amount of skeletal material excavated under the direction of Dr. A. V. Kidder from 1915 to 1924. It is now located in the Peabody Museum of Harvard. The specimen (Cat. No. 60, 280) was a female, aged 45 to 49, from Pecos Pueblo, New Mexico. It is thought to belong to Glaze IV time period, which would date it about A.D. 1600. This would not only be post-Columbian but also post-Spanish. According to Hooton's *Indians of Pecos Pueblo*, the Spanish first visited the Pecos Village in 1540 under the leadership of Francisco Coronado. The specimen had a "degenerative arthritis deformans of the right shoulder joint and Pott's disease (?) or spondylitis deformans."

This writer has not seen the specimen, but from the photograph pictured in Hooton's book it appears that there is involvement of six vertebrae firmly fused together with only a slight deformity. The possibility is more likely that this was a severe arthritis rather than tuberculosis. Dr. Hooton states that in an examination of 503 Pecos Pueblo skeletons it was noted that 13.2 percent had "spondylitis deformans" (arthritis of the spine).

Case 4 (Valcarcel and Garcia-Frias). In 1940 Dr. Garcia-Frias, Medical Director of the Clavegoya Sanitarium of Jauja, Peru, reported a case of what was thought to be tuberculosis in a Peruvian mummy. Mummies found in a certain arid area of Peru are dehydrated and actually contain flesh, skin, hair, and organs in a dried state; and by a process of hydration the tissues can be brought back to some resemblance of their original histology. This particular mummy was named Jorobado (meaning hunchback) and was supplied to Dr. Garcia-Frias by the National Museum of Archaeology of Lima, Peru. The roentgenogram showed marked spinal kyphosis and compensating lordosis. From the ninth dorsal vertebra through the first lumbar, there was destruction of the bodies and fusion. Histologic studies of the hydrated lungs showed a large amount of fibrous tissue in the right apex. Dr. Garcia-Frias concluded that the combination of spine and lung disease showed that tuberculosis is the most likely diagnosis, and this writer agrees, although other conditions are not completely ruled out.

The mummy, Jorobado, was pronounced to be prehistoric by Dr. Valcarcel, Department of Anthropology, University of San Marcos, Lima, Peru, and his co-workers from Cuzco. However, a pre-Columbian date is difficult to establish in certain instances because there is no distinct dividing line between pre- and post-Columbian. For a considerable time after the discovery of America, many Peruvian Indians retained the same customs, used the same materials, and lived in the same manner as had their ancestors for years before America was discovered by the European.

Dr. Garcia-Frias reported on two other mummies studied by the hydration method: one had calcium deposits in hilar and mesenteric lymph nodes and the other had pleural adhesions. It is the opinion of the author that neither of the findings could justify a diagnosis of tuberculosis.

Case 5 (Requena, Dupouy, and Cruxent). "The first unmistakable evidence of pre-Columbian tuberculosis in America" is a statement of Dr. Antonio Requena when describing a diseased human vertebra found in January, 1945, by Dr. Requena, Walter

Dupuoy, and Jose Maria Cruxent. There are two questions that should be answered in this case: Is the specimen pre-Columbian, and is the pathology typical of tuberculosis?

In a personal communication, Walter Dupouy kindly submitted a large amount of additional information regarding the age of the specimen. The diseased vertebra came from the El Palito Archaeologic Site, State of Carobobo, Venezuela. Although no carbon dating has yet been applied to the El Palito Site, other sites of the same age determined through comparison of styles and materials have been submitted to carbon 14 analysis. Dupouy refers to a monograph, *An Archaeological Chronology of Venezuela*, written by J. M. Cruxent and Irving Rouse (1958). The archaeology of Venezuela was divided into five periods and the dates for each period were determined by various methods, including radiocarbon analysis.

According to the authors of that monograph, El Palito existed for a long span of time from late in Period II through Period III. Period II dated from 1050 B.C. to A.D. 350 and Period III from A.D. 350 to A.D. 1150. Any material found in El Palito would then date long before Columbus discovered Venezuela in 1498.

In regard to whether the specimen can be diagnosed as tuberculous, the following is quoted from Requena (1945): "Almost all of the internal portions of the bodies of the tenth and eleventh thoracic vertebrae are completely destroyed, leaving a large cavity covered by a thin shell of bone. This cavity is connected to a large fistulous tract opening on the surface of the body of the tenth thoracic vertebra."

A photograph included in the article shows the posterior view of the tenth and eleventh thoracic vertebrae. The caption under the photograph stated: "The posterior surface, viewed from above, of the 10th and 11th dorsal vertebrae. We see on the posterior surface of the 10th, the exterior posterior opening of the fistula." Without seeing the specimen it is unfair to draw any conclusions; but, according to Requena's description and the accompanying photo-

graph, there are two features atypical of spinal tuberculosis: (1) failure of the collapse of the diseased vertebra to create an angular deformity, and (2) the fistulous tract, described and pictured in the photograph, opening posteriorly, would occur very rarely in tuberculosis involving the lower thoracic vertebrae. Tuberculosis could be the cause of this pathology but it does not seem typical enough to justify the statement: "the first *unmistakable* evidence of pre-Columbian tuberculosis in America."

Cases 6, 7, and 8 (Ritchie). In September, 1952, three cases of suspicious spinal tuberculosis from New York State were reported by Dr. William A. Ritchie. Each case came from a separate Indian culture. All three are in the possession of the Rochester Museum of Arts and Sciences. According to Dr. Ritchie, there is no doubt of the pre-Columbian origin of all three. The actual specimen or the photographs and the roentgenograms were submitted for opinions as to diagnosis to 17 different medical specialists, including pathologists, orthopedic surgeons, radiologists, and several physicians interested in prehistoric pathology.

"The first specimen, Cat. No. A.P. 526 (Plate 29,B), was excavated in 1938 in a cemetery of flexed burials, Livingston County, New York, by William Ritchie and Charles Wray. It was an adult female between 26 and 30 years of age. It belonged to the prehistoric Iroquois occupation and would date about A.D. 1200.

"The lower 7 thoracic and all lumbar vertebrae, a total of 12, were involved in a destructive process. Necrosis of the bodies of the tenth, eleventh and twelfth thoracic vertebrae resulted in approximately a 90-degree angular deformity. There is firm fusion of the lower thoracic vertebrae and another partial fusion of the third and fourth lumbar. There are indications of multiple drainage canals involving the bodies, and pedicles and articular facets and erosion of anterior body surfaces suggest a large perivertebral abscess enveloping the entire dorsal column."

Catalog No. A.P. 529 was a skeleton of an adult male, 40 years of age, found in Munroe County, New York, by Ritchie and Wray. It belonged to the Owasco culture, which is thought to date somewhere between A.D. 500 and A.D. 1200. Ritchie describes this specimen as showing "a profound lesion which has destroyed the centra of the vertebral bodies of most of the thoracic segments of the spine, producing a kyphosis of slightly less than 90 degrees. The remnants, together with the lumbar vertebral bodies, have undergone firm fusion. A marked atrophy of the anterior lumbar bodies may have resulted from the pressure of a thick, walled-off abscess in the abdomen. Sinus formation and a slight amount of regenerated bone are also present."

Catalog No. A.P. 530, the third specimen described by Ritchie, was found by relic hunters in 1938 in Seneca County, New York. The specimen consisted of seven ankylosed thoracic vertebrae. The rest of the skeleton was not saved. Ritchie checked the site and ascertained that it was pre-Columbian in time and belonged to the Middle Point Peninsula culture (date about 2,000 years ago). He states: "The specimen consists of 7 thoracic vertebrae, ankylosed into a solid piece which exhibits a complete kyphoscoliosis. The neural arch structure, both facets and laminae, are fused to the degree that they have completely lost their identity. The spinous and transverse processes are intact except for postmortem destruction, and the vertebral canal is patent throughout. Fine bony trabeculations extend throughout the fused bodies."

The medical specialists, in evaluating these three cases, were not unanimous in their opinions. The majority favored the diagnosis of tuberculosis as likely for all three but, as expected, there was considerable disagreement. The difficulties of diagnosing tuberculosis from the dried specimen alone are obvious. Not only is there a great scarcity of proven dried specimens of tuberculosis of the spine, but many cases of tuberculosis in the past, diagnosed principally roentgenographically, have never been verified. The one atypical finding common to all three of Ritchie's specimens is the extensive involvement (in A.P. 526, 12 vertebrae; in A.P. 529, possibly 17; and in A.P. 530, at least 7).

Case 9 (Plate 29,C) (O'Bannon and Lichtor). This specimen was discovered by Lloyd Gordon O'Bannon during a series of excavations undertaken by the Clarksdale Chapter of the Tennessee Archaeological Society (O'Bannon 1957). The skeleton came from Montgomery County, Tennessee, Site M.T. 17. It is from a stone box burial and belongs to the Mississippian culture which existed in this area, according to Professor Thomas M. N. Lewis, sometime from A.D. 1000 to A.D.1600. The specimen is an adult; the sex could not definitely be determined. The description by Dr. Joseph Lichtor, orthopedic surgeon (Lichtor and Lichtor 1957), is as follows: The specimen, the skull and spine of which have been accepted for inclusion in the National Collections of the Smithsonian Institution, consists of a kyphotic thoracolumbar spine made up of 7 vertebrae, the tenth thoracic through the fourth lumbar vertebrae. Except for the proximal one, all the intervening intervertebral discs have been destroyed. The vertebral bodies have collapsed and fusion has taken place. The intervertebral facet joints and neural arches are similarly affected. Throughout the kyphotic curve, the spinal canal is patent and undistorted. The pathological changes are characteristic of spinal tuberculosis."

The involvement of 7 vertebrae and the excessive bony regeneration are certainly not typical of the pathology caused by tuberculosis.

Case 10 (Judd and Stewart). This is a child burial from Pueblo Bonito, excavated by Neil Judd in 1947. The date is A.D. 828-1130. The specimen is now on display in an exhibit in the Armed Forces Medical Museum. There is partial destruction of bodies of T-12 and L-2, with almost complete destruction of L-1. There is fusion of the bodies of these three vertebrae. In addition, there is a 45-degree angular deformity.

This case is quite typical of tuberculosis with destruction of vertebral bodies, angular deformity, and little bone regeneration.

Case 11 (Stewart). This specimen was excavated in 1955 at Nanjemoy Creek, Maryland, by Dr. Dale Stewart. The culture is Algonquin. The date is prior to 1608. No white contact material was found. All the lumbar vertebrae are involved and there are angulation deformities. Regeneration of bone is a prominent feature with complete fusion of L-1, 2, and 3. The specimen is on display at the Armed Forces Medical Museum, Washington, D. C.

This case could be tuberculosis, but the amount of regeneration of bone is atypical. It also is probably not pre-Columbian.

Case 12 (Nash). This case is located in the burial mound at Chucalissa, a state park near Memphis, Tennessee. The burial is one of many excavated by the Parks Archaeologist, Charles Nash, and is permanently on exhibit. It is a male, age 30 to 33, and belongs to the Mississippian culture. Five radiocarbon dates have been obtained on this site, ranging from A.D. 1027 to 1617. This burial is in the upper part of the mound, which suggests that it probably belongs closer to the 1600 date. Although this is pre-white contact, it is probably not pre-Columbian. Disease, newly introduced, could travel faster than the actual settlement of the territory by the whites.

This specimen comes very close to being typical tuberculosis. Two vertebrae are involved. The bodies of T-7 and 8 have apparently been completely destroyed and are not present. T-7 and 8 are fused at their inferior and superior articular processes, giving an acute angular deformity (about 45 degrees). There is very little, if any, evidence of new bone formation.

Case 13 (Plate 29,E). In the early 1930's a farmer, Glen McGirr, was digging for relics at the Crable Site, Fulton County, Illinois. Knowing that Don Dickson was interested in bone pathology, Mr. McGirr took to Dickson Mounds anything he found which appeared abnormal. One of the specimens was a conglomeration of 10 vertebrae, T-5 through L-1, all firmly fused together. The angle of deformity was about 160 degrees. (See photograph). The verte-

brae were firmly fused through the bodies, neural arches, and transverse processes. There was tremendous regeneration of bone. The neural canal was patent. No other parts of the skeleton were saved so it is impossible to tell the sex and age. However, the specimen appears to be from a small adult. Crable is a Late Mississippian village site and cemetery. It appears to have been occupied by many people for a relatively short period of time. Three carbon 14 dates have been obtained by Dr. H. R. Crane, University of Michigan.

Samples M-553, M-550, and M-554 were assigned the chronologic dates: A.D. 1330, A.D. 1360, and A.D. 1420.

The most prominent feature of this specimen is the extreme deformity and tremendous regeneration of bone. Involvement of 10 vertebrae and massive bone regeneration would not favor a diagnosis of tuberculosis. Many burials have been excavated by individual diggers at Crable. No other similar specimens have been found.

Case 14 (Plate 29,F). This is Burial 6, Emmons Cemetery, Fulton County, Illinois, excavated by Dan F. Morse and Merrill Emmons. It is a male, 36 years of age. The normal height should be 5 feet, 6 inches, but, due to the deformity and telescoping of the spine, the individual would be about 6 to 8 inches shorter. The culture is Middle Mississippian, with definite "old village" influence. No carbon dates have been reported as yet, but from the associated artifacts, the approximate date would be A.D. 1200 to 1300. All 5 lumbar and the lower 3 thoracic vertebrae are involved in a twisted, compressed mass of bone destruction and massive regeneration. The fifth lumbar is pathologically fused to the sacrum. There are many holes in the anterior surfaces of bodies of the involved vertebrae, suggesting multiple fistulas. There is a 45-degree angular deformity which probably was compensated by positioning. The most prominent feature besides the bony regeneration is the telescoping of the vertebrae. Although the neural arches are fused, as are the transverse processes, the spinal canal is patent.

The features that would be contrary to diagnosis of tuberculosis are the extensive involvement (8 vertebrae and sacrum) and the large amount of bony regeneration.

Case 15 (Plate 29,D). This specimen was given to Don Dickson by Rod Hiles, a retired construction worker. It was found near the surface in a Hopewell Mound near Frederick, Illinois; but, since it was not scientifically excavated, its culture and date cannot be accurately determined. The reason for its being dug was that the mound was located on a hillside which had been optioned by a contractor who intended to use the ground for fill to repair a levee. No artifacts were found with this skeleton or with any of the other skeletons found buried near the surface. However, the two tombs located at the bottom of the mound contained Hopewell material, and many examples of Late Woodland and Hopewell pottery were found scattered in the mound fill and in the immediate surrounding area. The author's guess is that the skeleton most likely belonged to a late Hopewell culture.

Most of the skeleton was present. The skull was badly crushed. The left tibia, part of one fibula, an ulna, and most of the bones of the feet and hands were missing, as were the first cervical and the eleventh and twelfth thoracic vertebrae. It was the skeleton of a young male about 25 years of age, height 5 feet, 3½ inches (possibly 2 inches less because of deformity). All thoracic and lumbar vertebrae except L-5 showed a moderate-to-severe amount of osteoarthritis as evidenced by lipping; bony spurs and a bony bridge joined L-3 and 4. There was a severe destructive osteomyelitis involving the bodies of thoracic vertebrae 5 through 10. Almost all of the body of T-8 was completely destroyed, with partial destruction of T-7 and about three-quarters of T-9. Two small sinus openings were seen on the anterior surface of T-10. The neural canal was patent. Small nodules were seen on the surface of the bodies of T-5 through T-11, indicating a moderate amount of bony regeneration with bone destruction, while there was a fusion of the bodies of T-8 and 9, involving a small part of the transverse

processes. A 45-degree angular kyphosis was caused by the collapse of the bodies of T-8 and 9.

With such an extensive destructive lesion, death must have occurred rather rapidly. Bony regeneration as seen by the nodules and fusion of two of the vertebrae must have occurred early, suggesting that this was an acute severe type of osteomyelitis and of short duration. However, it certainly could have been caused by tuberculosis. It is unfortunate that scientific excavation techniques were not followed. Since it would seem that the individual was either Late Hopewell or post-Hopewell Woodland, the probable date would fall between A.D. 200 and A.D. 1000.

Case 16 (Allison, Mendoza, and Pezzia). In 1973 a case of tuberculosis existing in an 8- to 10-year-old male Peruvian mummy was reported. The date (A.D. 700) and culture (Nazia Culture of Southern Peru) was established by associated grave goods and carbon dating of muscle tissue. Pathology (x-ray and autopsy) revealed erosion of the first, second, and third lumbar vertabrae with an associated psoas abscess and multiple nodules involving the lungs, pleura, liver, and right kidney. These nodules contained acid fast bacilli. In a personal communication (July 14, 1976), Dr. Marvin J. Allison writes:

In regard to your question on additional cases of tuberculosis in pre-Columbian America we have the following:

1. A healed primary in a Huari girl who died of collagen disease. No bacilli. A.D. 925.

2. A healed Potts disease in an Inca woman. Time about of the conquest; could be before or after.

3. A young girl with a radiographic lesion in lumbar area compatible with early tuberculosis. Unfortunately organs in body cavity are not in condition to do any studies. Area of lesions was negative for bacteria.

In the original article concerning Case 16 there is the following quotation (Allison et al. 1973):

The case presented herein should conclusively end this dispute and remove all doubt that tuberculosis did exist in the Department of Inca in Southern Peru, South America, hundreds of years before the coming of any European to the Americas.

The author agrees, but still if a contagious disease like tuberculosis was present in overcrowded prehistoric populations, which did exist in many parts of the Americas, then there should be many more cases of suspect tuberculosis than have been found to date.

Summary of Cases. A series of 16 cases of spinal disease occurring in the American Indian is presented. Of the 16, one (Case 16) established beyond a doubt that tuberculosis did exist in an 8- to 10-year-old Peruvian mummy. Only four of the remaining (Cases 4, 10, 12 and 15) could be considered typical enough to give a strong presumption of spinal tuberculosis, and in one of these cases (Case 12 Nash) a pre-Columbian date is not certain. Even in these four, other diseases could have caused the same changes. In most of the remaining 11 cases, tuberculosis could have been the cause but certain features throw some doubt on such a diagnosis.

Treponema Infection

Syphilis and yaws produce similar pathological changes in bones (Hackett 1951; Williams 1935). It is difficult to compare the two because different degrees of destruction and sclerosis will occur in the various stages of both diseases. The principal differences are that congenital syphilis, in the very young, causes an osteochondritis (Karsner 1955: 798) and yaws does not (Hackett 1951). Joint involvement is rare in syphilis–and is supposed to be nonexistent in yaws (Williams 1935). Also, yaws is restricted to the Tropics (Stewart and Spoehr 1952).

The outstanding characteristics of both diseases are these (see Ritvo 1955, Pugh 1958; Karsner 1955; Cole et al., 1955; and Hackett 1951):

(1) A gummatous periostitis and osteitis principally affecting the shafts of the long bones, most frequently the tibiae.

(2) New bone formation on the surface of the diseased areas; when it occurs on the anterior portion of the tibia, it may result in "saber shin" deformity.

(3) Thickening of the cortex, sometimes causing localized swelling of the bone and/or a narrowing of the medullary cavity.

(4) Occasionally a gumma extends into the marrow space. Sequestra are rare.

(5) In the skull the most frequently involved bones are the frontal and the parietal. Here there can be a periosteal osteitis sometimes located in the outer table only; but occasionally a gumma can produce a large area of destruction.

(6) Both yaws and syphilis can cause a destructive lesion of the face, resulting in destruction of the nose, palate and the anterior alveolar area (gangosa). (See Williams 1935; and Knaggs, 1926).

The following two cases of possible treponema infection in prehistoric America are presented with the help of Don Brothwell, British Museum of Natural History; Dr. A. J. Novotny, orthopedic surgeon, Peoria, Illinois; Larry Conrad, archaeologist, formerly with the Illinois State Museum; Dr. L. C. Burt, veterinarian, Petersburg, Illinois; and Alan Harn, artist-archaeologist, Dickson Mounds Museum.

CASE 1.
Location: Roger Briney Farm, SW1/4 of NE1/4, Sec. 1, Hickory Twp., Schuyler Co., Ill.
Excavated by: Dr. L. C. Burt
Culture Affiliation: Mississippian (probable date A.D. 1200–1400).
Disposition: Dickson Mounds Museum.

In conducting "pasture improvement" in the year 1960, Roger Briney uncovered some portions of skeletons on top of a high hill on his farm overlooking Route 100 in Schuyler County, Illinois. This location has been designated as being in the "Rose Mound Group" surveyed and excavated in 1928 by University of Illinois archaeologists. The Rose Mounds consisted of 19 mounds, which were divided into separate groups. The exact number of the mound from which this burial came could not be determined; but apparently it came from the second group, designated as Mounds 7 through 19. The cultural affiliations of the Rose Mounds, as reported in *Transactions of the American Philosophical Society,* November, 1941, were principally Middle Mississippian. It is further apparent from this report and description of associated artifacts that one of the mounds (No. 13) contained both Mississippian and Late Archaic (Red Ocher) remains.

According to Dr. L. C. Burt who excavated and removed the skeleton designated as Case 1, this skeleton was in an extended position and was partially covered with "red stain"; associated with the burial was a stone Mississippian elbow pipe, a long bone needle and a single shell bead. Also, lying on the chest of the burial was a skeleton of a small infant, age about one month. Several feet of soil from the top of the ridge had been removed by farm equipment. This skeleton, according to Dr. Burt, was approximately 5 feet farther down, making the total depth at least 7 feet from the 1960 surface.

In the summer of 1966, Don Brothwell and the author had the privilege of examining and photographing this skeleton at Petersburg, Illinois. Later the author acquired the specimen and it will be permanently housed at the Dickson Mounds Museum.

The following description is by Don Brothwell.

The skeleton is complete except that one thoracic vertebra was missing. It is a male, aged 30–40 years.

Skull and Teeth

```
            A
    R     C C                                R
R   8 7 6 5 4 3 X X  │  X X 3 4 5 6 7 8
    ─────────────────┼─────────────────  L
    8 7 6 5 4 3 2 1  │  1 2 3 4 5 6 X 8
            C C
            A
```

A—abscess at root
C—cavity
X—tooth lost antemortem
R—tooth reduced in size

The teeth are in fair condition, demonstrating very little attrition. The upper four incisors are missing, along with the adjacent alveolar area. The palate is perforated, showing pitting and irregularity.

The front view of the skull shows considerable nasal destruction, including the anterior alveolar area, and extends up to and including the nasal bones. Part of the frontal bone is also involved, showing irregular pits and sinus formation. The margins of the nasal orifice are rounded and smoothed by an unsuccessful attempt at repair following an inflammatory reaction. The basisphenoid shows inflammation and the inner part of the nose appears to be destroyed. The margins of the maxillary sinuses (within nose) display some reaction, but there is no evidence of change within the sinuses (Plate 30,A; Plate 31,A,B).

Postcranial Skeleton (Plate 30,B; Plate 31,C, D,E)

The postcranial skeleton shows various damages, mainly in the long bones, and is generally restricted to the shafts. The bones involved are as follows:

Both tibiae. The shafts (especially the left) show an ulcerative osteomyelitis of the kind seen in yaws and syphilis (i.e., of a treponemal type). The anterior portions of the shafts are particularly affected. There is no involvement of the joints.

Right femur. The distal articular end is the only portion involved. This shows a spreading periostitis which involves a small portion of the shaft. The patellar area of the joint surface shows erosion.

Right patella. The posterior surface has some small raised areas of irregularity.

Right scapula. The disease is limited to a small area reaction on the acromion process.

Right ulna. The upper third of the shaft and the anterior olecranon notch is involved in deep ulceration and minimal regenerative nodulation. The joint is not involved.

Both humeri. The disease is restricted to the distal fourth. The left is more involved than the right. The involvement shows a destructive ulceration with irregular nodulation.

Left clavicle. Only one clavicle is involved. The ulcerative disease is restricted mainly to the distal half.

The *pelvis, rib, hand,* and *foot bones* are normal. There are no vertebral changes except for slight to severe osteoarthritis.

Estimation of disability

Physical disability would be mild to moderate, depending on the amount of pain in the affected bone and the amount, if any, of generalized toxicity due to the disease. Since the joints are not involved, there would be no limitation of movement. None of the bones show any porosis, indicating the Indian was physically active up to the time of death. The cosmetic disability was quite pronounced because of the large destructive ulceration of his face (gangosa). The presence of a small infant in the same grave might indicate that this adult, unable to carry on his share of the labor usually performed by men, may have been assigned a woman's work.

CASE 2.

Location: Thompson Site, SW1/4 of SE1/4 of NW1/4, Sec. 15, Banner Twp., Fulton Co., Illinois.
Excavated by: Larry Conrad, Illinois State Museum.
Culture Affiliation: Early Mississippian (probable date A.D. 1000).
Disposition: Dickson Mounds Museum.

In the summer of 1962, Larry Conrad excavated a mound on the Thompson farm in Fulton County, Illinois. Twenty-nine burials were excavated. From the associated artifacts the culture was determined to be Early Mississippian because of the presence of "old village" material. Most of the burials were in a flexed position, a fact that tends to support the early A.D. 1000 date. Records and photographs were taken of the excavation as work proceeded. Case 2 was a flexed burial. It was cleaned off and prepared for photography. Mr. Conrad stated that it was apparently a complete skeleton *in situ*. During the absence of the crew, two small boys removed the skeleton. Later it was recovered from one of their homes. Unfortunately some entire bones and some portions of other bones were missing and could not be located.

The following is a description of T-6 (Case 2) by Dr. A. J. Novotny.

The skeleton was a male, age about 35.

Skull.

Over one-half of the right side of mandible and maxilla are lost postmortem.

Teeth show moderate attrition.

$$R \frac{/\ /\ /\ /\ /\ /\ /}{/\ /\ /\ 5\ 4\ 3\ 2\ 1} \Bigg| \frac{/\ 2\ 3\ 4\ 5\ 6\ 7\ 8}{1\ 2\ /\ 4\ 5\ 6\ 7\ X} L$$

X—tooth lost antemortem
/—tooth lost postmortem

The anterior surface of the frontal bone is involved, showing roughening and subperiosteal thickening. There are several small holes located above the eye sockets, with some slight surrounding erosion. These holes involve only the outer table (Plate 30,D; Plate 31,W).

Postcranial Skeleton

Some of the bones of the postcranial skeleton are missing postmortem. All uninvolved long bones present show moderate porosis. The following bones are involved:

Tibiae. The right is heavier than the left. This is due to hypertrophy of the proximal two-thirds. There are many tiny pits located on the medial surface of the proximal two-thirds. The left tibia appears normal except for some minimal cortical pitting in the medial aspect of the upper fourth.

Fibulae. Right fibula is missing. The left fibula is normal.

Ribs. The ribs are fragmentary and many are missing. Portions of six ribs show thickened irregular surfaces with bone destruction and some nodulations.

Right clavicle. There is enlargement of the lateral half of the right clavicle with moderate destruction plus some regenerative nodulation. (The left clavicle is missing.)

Right ulna. There is enlargement of the upper third of the shaft. The medial surface shows pitting and irregularity where there are two sinus holes measuring 3 mm. in diameter. The joint surface shows lipping but the disease does not involve the joint (Plate 31,X).

Left ulna. The left ulna (lower half missing postmortem) is normal except for lipping of the elbow joint margins.

Right radius. Minimal similar changes in the proximal end. (The left radius is missing postmortem.)

Right humerus. The same disease process involves the distal half and consists of irregular surfaces, sinus formation and cortical erosion. There is perforation of the olecranon fossa (congenital) with the cortical erosion extending into the fossa. The entire bone seems shortened. There appears to have been an old fracture (now well healed) involving the distal third with 20-degree varus angulation. This fracture may be pathological or could be entirely unrelated to the main disease (Plate 31,Y).

Left femur. Heavier than the right. The distal one-half is swollen with an irregular anterior surface, pitting and new bone formation. There is a 1 cm. hole at the lower fourth on the anterior surface, with several deeper sinus tracts (Plate 31,Z).

Right femur. The lower one-half is thickened and sclerosed. All surfaces of the lower one-half of the shaft are irregular. There is a 5 mm. sinus tract located at the upper end of the diseased portion on the anterior surface.

Sacrum and greater trochanter of right femur. On the dorsal aspect of the sacrum, in the midline involving the fourth, fifth and sixth segments, is a bony abnormality characterized by a slight bone destruction and a predominant bony proliferation forming multiple nodules from 1 mm. to 1 cm. in diameter. A similar lesion is found at the lateral aspect of the greater trochanter of the right femur. These two areas are different in character from the disease process in the other bones, and involve points of subcutaneous bony prominence and are common sites of decubitus ulceration (Plate 30,E).

Seven thoracic and five lumbar vertebrae are available for examination. All show mild lipping. There is a slight wedging of the second lumbar. Both the right and left innominate bones are normal. Only a few tarsals and other foot bones are present and show no abnormalities.

Microscopic Section

Karl R. Sohlberg, M.D., Chairman, Dept. Pathology, St. Francis Hospital, Peoria, Illinois.

Rib: "Grossly, there appears to be thickening, particularly of the flatter surface toward one end. Sections were taken both from this end and from the end which appeared normal. We were quite surprised at how little decalcification was required to prepare this for sectioning.

"As might be expected, the histologic preparation shows a major degree of artifact, presumably because of chemical action in the soil from many years of burial. Nevertheless, those portions of bone which retained fairly good morphologic characteristic appear quite regular, particularly with respect to the Haversian systems. I am unable to state with certainty the nature of the defects in the cortical surface noted grossly, since their margins are badly altered from the long exposure.

"I do not believe that I am able to define any pathologic process in the material under study, and more specifically, there is nothing here that suggests Paget's Disease" (Plate 30,C).

Roentgenologic Interpretation

R. S. Malcolm, M.D., Staff Roentgenologist, Methodist Hospital, Peoria, Illinois.

"X-rays of this case include films of long bones, ribs, sternum, clavicle and skull. Almost all of the bones appear to be involved by similar process. The shafts of the long bones reveal considerable cortical thickening and sclerosis, apparently mainly on the external aspect; but there is also evidence of some endosteal proliferation so that the medullary cavity apparently is encroached on in some instances. A transverse section of one of the long bones reveals this to be the case. There are scattered areas of rarefaction apparently representing areas of destruction. The lateral view of the skull reveals apparently minor involvement of the outer table of the frontal bone with some cortical irregularity, rarefaction and associated sclerosis noted in this region.

"The findings are compatible with those seen in late congenital or acquired syphilis."

Estimation of Disability

The porosis of the long bones was probably the result of physical inactivity. The changes on the sacrum and greater trochanter would require months to develop and suggest a long period of recumbency. The disability must have been severe for a long period of time, indicating not only considerable tolerance for his illness by people in his community but would necessitate a great amount of attention and care.

Comment

In summary these two cases represent a disseminated inflammatory disease of bone wherein there are adjacent areas of the involved bone and adjacent entire bones that appear normal. The disease is characterized by a periostitis, osteitis and osteomyelitis, the predominating lesions being periostitis and osteitis. There is both bony destruction and bony proliferation, with multiple sinus tract formation. The process is principally located on the diaphysis and metaphysis with little or no joint involvement. In both cases there is an osteitis limited to the outer table of the frontal bone and in one case there is an extensive destruction of the skeletal structures of the mid-face.

Among those conditions that should be considered in the differential diagnosis are: chronic purulent osteomyelitis; chronic sclerosing osteomyelitis of Garré; tuberculosis; Paget's disease; and mycotic infection.

Purulent osteomyelitis can reasonably be ruled out because of no joint involvement, absence of evidence of sequestra, and the fact that the predominant lesion is not destructive osteomyelitis but a periostitis.

Chronic sclerosing osteomyelitis (Myerding 1944) is usually not so widely distributed and the presence of abscesses and evidence of sinus formation in the two cases would indicate that some pus was present.

Tuberculosis creates destruction of the bone with little or no regeneration; and in such a generalized distribution it would certainly affect its favorite site—the joints.

Case 1 does not present any features suggesting Paget's. In Case 2, Paget's is ruled out microscopically.

Mycotic disease usually affects the bones by direct extension from soft tissue abscesses. Multiple involvement does occur rarely, especially in coccidiodal infection (Benninghoren and Miller 1942).

Those interested in paleopathology must face the frustrating fact that the same disease can cause different patterns of bone pathology and many different diseases are capable of producing the same pattern. In clinical experience, using all available diagnostic paraphernalia the declared diagnosis is not always the correct one. Undoubtedly, these two cases most closely resemble treponema infection.

The most impressive evidence that syphilis was of American origin is that the great epidemics in the Old World occurred at the time of or soon after the discovery of America by Columbus. Failure to find prehistoric skeletal pathology resembling "Charcot's joints" and aneurysmal distortion (erosion of thoracic vertebrae) is the best argument against the American origin of syphilis. Perhaps syphilis did exist in the pre-Columbian New World, but not in the same form as we know it today (Morse 1969).

Paget's Disease (Osteitis Deformans)

Osteitis deformans is a bone disease of unknown etiology occurring in middle and old age and is more frequent in men than in women. Paget's can be widely distributed (polyostotic) or involve one (monostotic) or a few bones. Any or all bones in the body can be affected. Those most frequently involved are the pelvis, skull, vertebrae and femurs. In the natural history of Paget's there are usually three phases. The first phase is characterized by a destructive process which can be an expanding area of lysis with sharply demarcated borders between normal and diseased bone; and in the long bones, involvement may include the entire transverse diameter and ultimately the entire shaft. In the skull this localized area of destruction may be seen in the x-ray as a well-defined decrease in density called "osteoporosis circumscripta." The second phase begins almost immediately with deposition of new bone and the result is a combination of destruction and regeneration. The final phase, which may appear years later, is the so-called "healing stage," which means that the deposition of bone is the predominant characteristic.

The combination phase of Paget's disease is most frequently encountered and it is then that microscopic sections and the x-ray will show typical features. The pathology is characterized by an osteoclastic resorption of bone and a simultaneous osteoblastic regeneration of, at first, coarse vascular fibrous bone, which later becomes the site of deposition of lamellar bone. Both processes, destruction and regeneration, are going on at the same time and the end result is seen *microscopically* as many tiny segments of bone of various shapes and sizes, each surrounded by indefinite cement lines. This "mosaic pattern" gives the appearance of being highly disorganized. The Haversian canals can become large and the normal Haversian architecture, which can be seen in microscopic sections of many archaeological bone specimens, is lost.

This same pathology can cause changes in the x-ray, depending on the phase of the disease. In the long bones, this deposition of new bone can take on the appearance of linear trabeculae of increased density, separated by spaces of rarefaction sometimes being referred to as being "combed." Various degrees of bone destruction and localized areas of sclerosis appear, depending on the stage of advancement. The diseased portion of a bone can be greatly thickened due to both endostial and periostial formation of new bone and the medullary canal narrowed or obliterated. In the skull, the tables can be thickened, especially the outer table. The areas of new bone on the background of general porosis, plus irregular borders, have been described as "cotton wooly."

Other features of osteitis deformans are the deformities caused by bending and fractures. It has been emphasized that Paget's is not a generalized bone disease, as normal bone is always encountered at the edges of and between affected areas. Paget's has been known to be limited to only one bone throughout the life of an individual.

Dr. Alton K. Fisher (1935) reported a case of Paget's found by an archaeological field party of the Milwaukee Public Museum in 1929 in a prehistoric mound in Crawford County, Wisconsin. The specimen was fragmentary, consisting of both tibiae and a small portion of the lower jaw. The author has seen the gross specimens which are now located at the Milwaukee Public Museum. The jawbone appeared normal. Both tibiae were bowed and were slightly thickened. A longitudinal section of one tibia revealed that new bone deposition had caused considerable narrowing of the medullary canal. Fisher reports nothing about the microscopic appearance except an enlargement of the Haversian canals.

In March of 1968, Dr. Robert Ritzenthaler, Curator of Anthropology, Milwaukee Public Museum, sent the left tibia to the Armed Forces Institute of Pathology, Washington, D.C. The specimen was thoroughly examined by x-ray and microscopic sectioning. Dr. Lent Johnson (personal communication) reports that this was "not Paget's Disease." This experience emphasizes that archaeological Paget's should not be diagnosed except by positive x-ray and microscopic findings, and it creates some doubts concerning other reports of prehistoric Paget's.

Dr. Henri Stearns Denninger (1933) reports five cases of "Paget's" in prehistoric Indian skeletons excavated from mounds in the Illinois River Valley by the University of Chicago Archaeological Survey. Specimen 1, from Parker Heights Park, Quincy, Illinois, was in a poor state of preservation. It was considered prehistoric, but the culture was not determined. No age or sex was given. The bones showed an increase in size, some obliteration of the marrow cavities by spongy bone, bowing deformities and surface porosity. Specimen 2 was from Langford's (1927) Fisher Mound Group, near Joliet, Illinois (Late Mississippian Culture). This skeleton, a male 80 years old, consisted of the humeri, tibiae, fibulae and skull. The long bones showed similar changes as described in Specimen 1. The skull showed a thickened dense sclerotic calvarium, with the diploic architecture obliterated. Specimens 3, 4 and 5 were discovered in the summer of 1930 from Mounds F-13 and F-14, Fulton County, near Lewistown, Illinois. They were probably of Late Woodland culture. Specimen 3 was a female, aged 60. Specimen 4 was a male, aged 50. Both of these showed thickness of the skull bones, elevations and depressions over the frontal and occipital areas and a "solid, ivory-like appearance to the calvarium." The long bones were enlarged and there were "surface and hyperostotic changes." Specimen 5 was a male between 60 and 65. Only the distal half of the right tibia and the entire right fibula were affected. These showed rugged and porotic surfaces and some "sheets of fine spongy trabeculation" in the medullary cavity of the tibia. This indicates, according to the author, a monostotic form of "Paget's Disease." Microscopic examination apparently was not obtained on any of the five cases reported by Dr. Denninger.

Collins (1966) states that Paget's is almost nonexistent before the age of 40. After 40, the overall incidence is around 3 percent, with a sharp rise in incidence as the individual gets older. The scarcity of this disease in archaeological specimens could be accounted for by the fact that prehistoric man rarely reached the age in which Paget's is common.

CHAPTER 10

THE X-RAY

X-rays were discovered by William Konrad Roentgen in 1895, an accomplishment which came about after years of hard work on the part of many scientific investigators. This discovery was recognized immediately for its application to medical science and has been considered as one of the most important in medical history. X-rays are of value to the paleopathologist because they can show changes in the internal structure of the dried bone that are not apparent by gross examination of the specimen. Furthermore the x-rays of dried bone can be compared with abnormal films that have been clinically documented to have been caused by a specific disease entity. These documented films can be found in many publications and by the thousands in radiological laboratories. X-rays have also been used in looking for both bone and soft tissue pathology in dried and mummified specimens (Harris and Weeks 1973).

Nature

X-rays are electromagnetic radiations with a short wave length. A wave length is measured in Angstrom units, one Angstrom defined as 1/100,000,000th of a centimeter. Useful x-rays vary in wave length from 0.5 to 0.125 Angstroms and are about ten thousand times shorter than the wave length of visible light rays. They travel in straight lines from their originating point at 186,000 miles a second. Figure 8 shows the spectrum of electromagnetic radiations from the cosmic rays, which are the shortest, to the long electrical waves. X-rays are produced when a stream of electrons, flowing from the cathode (−) toward the anode (+) in a vacuum tube, strike a target in their path (Fig. 9). When this occurs, a great deal of heat is generated and, at the same time, x-rays are emitted, traveling in all directions from the target. Most of the

x-rays are absorbed by the casing of the vacuum tube except a few which escape through the window. The heat generated when the electrons strike the target is of concern to the radiologist because it can "burn out the tube." Several methods have been devised to decrease this possibility. The target can be mounted on a copper bar which is a good dissipater of heat. Water- or oil-cooling of the target area has been used. Some machines have a rotating anode in which the target becomes the rim of a revolving wheel, thus distributing the heat over a larger area and in this way contributing to the longevity of the x-ray tube. Every x-ray tube has a rating in regard to heat toleration. This depends on many factors including the melting point of the target and the cooling capacity of the tube. Limits of operation are influenced by time, kilovolts, and milliamperes. An increase of any or all of these will increase heat production. A tube can burn out by a single exposure above its rating or by several taken at close intervals without enough time between each exposure for sufficient cooling (Bloom et al. 1965: 34–37).

Properties

1. *Penetration* is the most significant property of x-rays. Their ability to penetrate mass is attributed to the shortness of their wave lengths. Whenever x-rays strike an object, some will be absorbed and some will penetrate. The amount of penetration depends on the thickness and density of the object and its atomic number. The higher the atomic number the more absorption and the less penetration. The effective atomic number of soft tissues is 7.4, and that of bone is 11.6; consequently, more rays will be absorbed by bone than by the soft tissues. Metals have high atomic numbers. Gold is 79, lead is 82,

60

etc. In metals very little if any penetration will occur.

2. *Photographic effects* of x-rays are similar to those of light since they cause the same changes in a photographic film. These changes in the silver salt emulsion can be made permanent by developing procedures. Those materials which are relatively non-penetrable because of high effective atomic numbers and/or of great thickness or density will show as white or light areas on a photographic negative (radiopaque); those objects such as air and soft tissues will show as black on the developed film (radiolucent); and between the two extremes varying shades of gray will result (intermediate).

3. *Fluorescence* (emission of visible light) will occur whenever x-rays strike certain substances, such as barium platinocyanide, calcium tungstate, etc. This property is of use in intensifying screens and fluoroscopy.

4. *Scattering* takes place whenever an x-ray beam strikes or is passing through matter, causing a reemission of secondary x-rays which then radiate in all directions from the point of contact. Avoidance of exposure to x-rays will not be accomplished by merely keeping out of the path of the x-ray beam coming from the machine because scattering may cause radiation contamination of the entire room. Just as the penetration power is increased in x-rays of shorter wave lengths, so is the incidence of scattering.

5. *Biological effects* of radiation include somatic and genetic damage. The effects of radiation are cumulative. The total dose ingested over a long period of time is just as dangerous as a large initial dose. Somatic damage includes skin erythemias, burns, and wounds that will not heal, skin cancer, leukemia and aplastic anemia. Since a large amount of x-ray exposure is required to cause somatic damage, the occurrence of these injuries in modern times is extremely rare because we have learned to employ adequate precautions so as to protect both the patient and the technicians in radiological laboratories (NCRP 1968). Genetic changes are a different matter since it is thought that damage will occur with small doses of radiation. Kinds of damage include (Graham 1973):

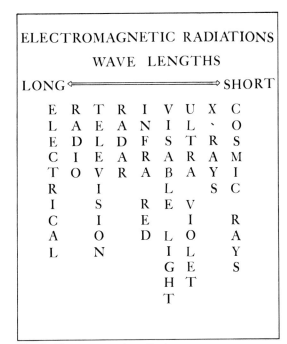

Fig. 8. Electromagnetic radiation spectrum.

(1) Death of cells if the dose is high enough. (Sex cells are very susceptible to radiation which may result in sterilization.)

(2) A breakdown of chromosomes causing malformations.

(3) A possible increase in mutations which could adversely affect the human race in future generations.

Not much is known about this third genetic damage, therefore, all unnecessary exposure to radiation should be avoided.

Protection

Since only bones and inanimate objects are x-rayed in a paleopathology laboratory, excessive radiation of the "patient" is of no concern. This enables the paleopathologists to use certain techniques that he might not care to use on living subjects, such as cardboard holders and long exposure times. The important concern is that all individuals who happen to be in the immediate vicinity, even in adjoining rooms, receive zero radiation. X-rays in departments of anthropology are to be considered nonmedical and should never be taken of living people, even in a supposed emergency. One of the better types of installation is where the tube portion of a portable

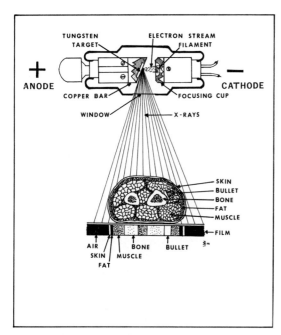

Fig. 9. The production of an x-ray.

machine—it could even be an older and cheaper model—is placed inside a box covered completely with lead sheeting, including the top and bottom. Lead sheets 2.5 mm in thickness would be more than adequate. A lead-covered door should be attached, and some sort of shelving on which to place specimens should be installed. The controls should be placed on the outside of the box and connected to the tube by a cable. If possible, a safety latch should be attached to the door so that the x-ray machine can not be turned on unless the door is closed. Before starting to use it, the equipment should be thoroughly tested by a radiology safety inspector. Possible leakage points to be checked are the door, the nails (should be lead-covered) used to attach the lead sheeting, and the point where the cable enters the box. Finally, a film badge or some type of monitoring device could be placed in the room at strategic positions to detect any leaks in the future.

Techniques

There are five principle variables that can be controlled by the technicians in an effort to get an adequate radiograph: the type of film, milliamperes (MA), kilovolts (KV), exposure time, and distance.

Films used should be the same as that used by medical radiologists usually denoted as "medical x-ray film." Special industrial films and high resolution negatives can be used for special projects.

Films are supplied by the manufacturer in two forms. In one form each film is individually wrapped in its own disposable paper or cardboard holder. Most dental and industrial films are supplied in this manner. In the other form, a number of films are packed in a box (usually 100). These must be loaded into holders or cassettes under darkroom conditions. For skeletal material, cardboard holders usually give the best detail. The film is placed in a lightproof paper envelope backed with cardboard. A thin layer of lead sheeting frequently is added to minimize back scattering from the table top. The second type of holder is a cassette containing intensifying screens. These are two sheets of a material coated with a fluorescent chemical such as calcium tungstate. The negative is placed between these two sheets. When the x-radiation strikes the cassette, the fluorescent chemical emits light which contributes to and intensifies the formation of the image on the photographic plate. The advantage is that the time can be decreased or the distance increased (Ross and Galloway 1963; Meschan 1959).

· *Milliampere* capacity varies in different models of x-ray machines and can be decreased or increased in most machines up to capacity. The technique of taking a film under certain conditions is sometimes expressed in milliampere seconds (MA-SEC.). For example, a chest film at 10 MA-Seconds on a machine that had a 10 MA capacity would require a one-second time exposure (the distance and KV remaining constant) while at 100 MA it would require 0.1 second to get a comparable film. Increasing the MA decreases the time and thus eliminating the bad effects of motion in a living subject. Since motion is of no concern to the paleopathologist, there is no need to install the more expensive equipment with a higher MA.

Kilovoltage is also a factor in getting a good result. When the KV is increased, x-rays of shorter wave lengths are produced thus increasing the power of penetration and also increasing the incidence of scattering. Scattering contributes to blurring of the image and loss of contrast. To decrease the KV, in order to decrease scattering, then the time of exposure must be increased to compensate for the decreased power of penetration.

Exposure time is dependent on the other variables. If the distance is increased the exposure time must be greater and vice versa. If the kilovoltage is decreased, then the time can be increased to compensate for loss of penetration. A greater milliamperage will permit a lesser time.

Distance from the tube to the film and from the subject to the film are important. Rays originating at the tube target and then leaving through the window travel in straight lines. The rays near the central portion of the beam strike the object to be photographed perpendicularly while those toward the periphery penetrate the specimen and come in contact with the film obliquely (Fig. 9). This results in distortion, loss of contrast and magnification. The shorter the distance from tube to film, the greater the magnification. It would appear that, in order to achieve minimum magnification, the tube-to-film distance should be in the neighborhood of six to eight feet. This is sometimes impractical because in order to compensate for the loss of intensity, the MA and/or the exposure time must be greatly increased, and this adjustment might be beyond the capacity of the machine. The intensity of the radiation at the photographic film is inversely proportional to the square of the distance used. If we double the distance, the time of exposure must be multiplied by four. Accuracy is desirable in certain procedures such as computerized osteometry (measuring bones) using radiographs, computerized profiles (Walker 1976), and print-outs of facial features (personal communication, Dr. Walker, University of Michigan). In these cases a magnification correction can be programed into the computer. This can be obtained by comparing actual distance between two bony landmarks on the specimen with the image on the radiograph. It is essential that a specific technique, in regard to distance and bone positioning, be employed so as to have comparable films. The subject-to-film distance should be as short as possible because any

significant increase here will also result in pronounced distortion and magnification. The percentage of magnification can be calculated using the following formula (Bloom et al. 1965: 106).

$$\frac{D}{D - d} - 1(100) = \% \text{ Mag.}$$

D = tube-film distance.
d = object-film distance.

One method of cutting down on distortion and blurring is the use of a Bucky, a frame supporting a number of thin parallel lead strips arranged in such a manner that the most oblique rays and some scattering will be absorbed by the sides of the strips. Only those rays passing through the spaces between the grids will come in contact with the film. The Bucky must move during the exposure so that no individual strip will be in one place long enough to cast its shadow on the radiograph. The disadvantage is that there must be an increase in time of exposure.

It is not possible to entirely eliminate distortion and magnification. If the object to be x-rayed is thick, such as a skull, then all features will be superimposed one on the other and registered as a single plane on the x-ray negative. Those features closest to the film will have the least distortion and magnification, and those farthest will have the most (Bloom et al. 1965: 105–107).

The technician should keep a record of the variables used to achieve satisfactory radiographs and make a chart for future reference. This chart should list all bones and, if applicable, different views of the same bone. The darkroom is important, but correct methods can best be learned by experience and personal instruction. Mistakes of the technician when taking the x-ray cannot be corrected in the darkroom. In other words, overexposure of the film can not be compensated by underdevelopment in the darkroom without loss of accuracy. One should remember that it is possible that an overexposure of a normal bone can give the impression of osteoporosis and underdevelopment can appear as sclerosis. Sometimes the interpreter will request variation in techniques so as to show internal structures in abnormal bone, for example, overexposure of sclerosis and under-

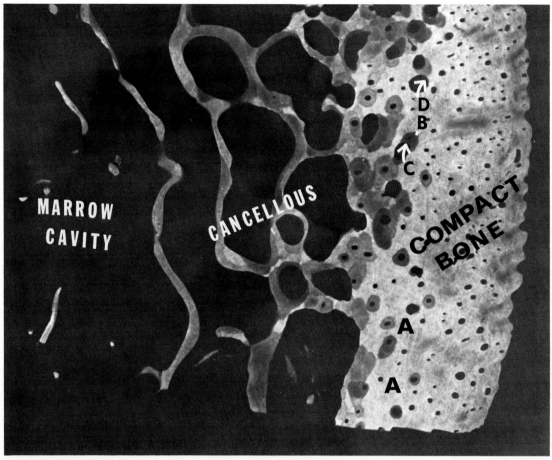

Fig. 10. Microradiograph (X50). Section of human femur. (A) Dense white is old well-mineralized bone; (B) Gray is new bone, i.e., recently formed and not yet well mineralized; (C) Surface undergoing active new bone formation (by apposition); (D) Surface undergoing active bone resorption. (Radiography courtesy of Dr. W. F. Enneking and Dr. Hans Burchardt, Department of Orthopedics, College of Medicine, University of Florida.)

exposure of porosis. The same could apply to bone that became demineralized because it had been in the ground too long.

In interpreting a radiograph, four factors should be taken into consideration (Enneking 1970) : (1) The distribution of the lesion in the skeleton, whether it is multiple or single, and its anatomic location; (2) The effect of the lesion on the bone, i.e., how much erosion and destruction is present; (3) The response of the bone to the lesion. Is the reactive bone proliferation zero to minimal as in multiple myeloma, small as in tuberculous osteitis, or great as in staphylococcal osteomyelitis? (4) Unique characteristics, such as the onion peel appearance in Ewings Sarcoma, the punched-out holes in multiple myeloma, the coarse trabecular pattern "combed appearance" in Paget's disease, etc.

Tomography

A technique of moving the x-ray tube and the film in opposite directions in such a manner that only one plane of the subject is in focus during the exposure is called tomography. All other areas of the subject in front and in back of the plane are out of focus and blurred out. The result is a radiograph of a thin slice of the subject. The x-ray tube is connected to the film carrier by a long lever which rotates on a pivot. By adjusting the pivot, a series of slices can be x-rayed. Other names have been applied to this procedure, such as planigraphy, laminagraphy and body section radiography. One of the most familiar uses of this technique is the detection of a cavity in a lung which is surrounded and hidden by a mass of inflamatory tissue. The value of this method in paleopathology is illustrated in Plate 37.

Microradiography

An excellent method of studying the physiology and pathology of bone is by microradiography. Using high resolution film, special equipment and decreasing the kilovoltage to a very low level, an x-ray of a thin bone section will reveal bone detail small enough to be seen through a microscope (Fig. 10) (Jowsey et al. 1965).

The technique used for preparing the specimen in Figure 10 is as follows: Embed a small piece of bone in methyl methacrylate. Slice with a milling machine or a diamond saw. Grind the slice down to 100 microns in thickness. X-ray, using 20 milliamperes and 20 kilovolts with approximately 5 to 20 minutes of exposure time. The distance (tube to film) was 20 cm. A special high resolution film (Kodak 50–20) was used.

CHAPTER 11

MICROSCOPIC ANALYSIS OF ARCHAEOLOGICAL BONE
DOUGLAS H. UBELAKER*

In recent years, skeletal biologists and paleo-pathologists have demonstrated an increasing reliance upon microscopic structure as a data source. Estimates of adult age at death made from thin sections of bone and teeth offer superior results to those produced from more conventional methods. Diagnoses of disease are occasionally enhanced when microscopic data are available. In addition, appraisals of nutrition and general health status may be improved from observations of bone micro-structure.

Historical Use of Microscope

Although the microscope is only recently becoming a standard tool in skeletal biology research, the history of its use in such studies extends back into the 19th century. As early as 1840, Sir Richard Owen examined microscopic structure in fossil teeth recovered by Agassiz. In a series of publications (1833–43) Agassiz himself described fossil dental comparative microstructure. In 1849, Quekett applied microscopy to fossil bone, and his later manual (1852) for the use of the microscope includes techniques for examining fossil bones and teeth.

Probably the first application to prehistoric man came in 1876 when Joseph Jones used thin sections to support his diagnosis of syphilis in prehistoric skeletons from Tennessee and Kentucky. Although his diagnosis is questionable, he noted, "When thin sections of these bones were carefully examined with the naked eye, and by the aid of magnifying glasses, portions were found resembling cancellous tissue from the enlargement and

irregular erosions of the Haversian canals, and increase in the number and size of the lacunae. . . ." (Jones 1876: 66).

Six years later, Broesike (1882) described the microstructure of a 200-year-old human tibia. He used a ground section to demonstrate that no organic material remained.

Beginning in 1910, Ruffer published a series of pioneer studies on paleopathology which concentrated primarily on Egyptian mummies. In this work he introduced histological technique to the examination of dessicated tissue (1921). Although his research concentrated on soft tissue, he did not ignore the skeleton. In 1910, he published microscopic descriptions of prehistoric urinary calculi associated with an Egyptian skeleton. In 1912, he described a spongy bone growth on the neck of an Egyptian femur. A microscopic examination of a section of the growth revealed "nothing peculiar." He also prepared decalcified thin sections of vertebrae and other bones with "spondylitis deformans," noting that the external lesions did not extend beyond superficial layers. In 1914, Ruffer added a description of internal features of an A.D. 250 Egyptian pelvic tumor. Using sections, Ruffer described in detail the internal cavities and trabeculae, although, due to the poor quality of the sections, he gleaned little microscopic information.

In 1918, Roy Moodie utilized sections to describe a lesion he called "osteoperiostitis" of a humerus of a fossil reptile. Later Moodie (1926) presented a detailed comparative histological study of normal and diseased fossil vertebrates. Moodie's texts on "The Antiquity of Disease" (1923a) and "Paleopathology" (1923b) frequently present microscopic data in describing osseous lesions on

---

* Associate Curator, Department of Anthropology, Smithsonian Institution.

fossil vertebrates. Prehistoric human bone sections are illustrated in describing a cranial "cauterization" (1923a:103) and an example of "cribra cranii interna."

Studies of fossil vertebrate comparative histology and skeletal disease have continued, with Enlow and Brown providing major contributions (1956, 1957, 1958). Ascenzi (1970) provided an excellent summary of publication in this area.

Histological studies of human mummy tissue since Ruffer's work have been numerous, with important contributions by Wilson (1927), Williams (1927, 1929a), Shaw (1938), Brothwell et al. (1969), Post and Daniels (1969), Sandison (1970), Yeatman (1971), Zimmerman et al. (1971), Zimmerman (1972), Allison et al. (1973), Allison, Pezzia, Hasegawa and Gerszten (1974), Allison, Pezzia, Gerszten and Mendoza (1974), Allison, Pezzia, Gerszten, Giffler, and Mendoza (1974), Allison and Gerszten (1975), Munizaga et al. (1975), Dalton et al. (1976), Gerszten, Allison, Pezzia and Klurfeld (1976), and Gerszten, Munizaga, Allison, and Klurfeld (1976).

Histological data have been utilized less frequently in prehistoric human bone research, but numerous examples since the work of Moodie are available. Weber (1927) utilized ground thin sections to document the gross histology of bones with possible syphilitic lesions. Weber (1927) and Williams (1929a) presented techniques for preparing sections of ancient bone. In addition, Williams (1929a,b) presented histological data on two immature Indian frontals with "symmetrical osteoporosis," documenting large cancellous spaces and destruction of the outer table. Sections of ribs of two other affected skeletons showed similar changes, suggesting to Williams that the skull condition reflected a general disorder of the bone marrow. Williams (1932), Nestmann (1928) and Michäelis (1930) all consulted microscopic data to support their diagnoses of syphilis in prehistoric bones. Williams (1932) provided a detailed discussion of histological changes produced by syphilis and other disorders. In his review of possible prehistoric examples of syphilis, Williams turned several times to histology for corroborative evidence. A section of a femur

from Pecos, New Mexico, revealed "structure of a periosteal osteophyte . . . confirmatory evidence for the syphilitic nature of the disease shown on the skull," (1932:934). Later, Williams used gross sections and decalcified stained thin sections to support a diagnosis of syphilis for material of Paracas, Peru (p.943–944), Cañete Valley, Peru (p.949–954), and Ohio (p.956–962).

In 1935, Denninger prepared a longitudinal section of a right tibia from Illinois considered to be pre-Columbian. The section revealed evidence which when correlated with surface observations and roentgenograms suggested a diagnosis of "adolescent luetic periostitis," (1935:204). Earlier, Denninger (1931:941–942) used microscopic data to support a diagnosis of osteitis fibrosa.

Similar conclusions were reached by Cole et al. (1955) following their examination of 57 skeletons from Arizona. Longitudinal sections from three individuals supported their diagnosis of syphilis and ruled out Paget's disease, "tuberculosis, actinomycosis, blastomycosis and yaws. . . ." (1955:234).

Recently, histological data has been used in research on prehistoric bone to suggest a diagnosis of syphilis (Goff:1967), rule out Paget's disease (Morse, 1967), document internal changes in degenerative joint disease (Ortner, 1968), describe bone loss due to osteoporosis (Van Gerven et al., 1970; Mielke et al., 1972; Van Gerven, 1973; Ericksen, 1973), compare lytic areas of possible myeloma (Berg, 1972), to document internal bone changes in a proposed example of generalized hyperostosis in a Peruvian mummy (Allison, Gerszten, Sotil and Pezzia, 1976), and to classify lesions of osteomyelitis and periostitis from prehistoric ossuaries in Ontario, Canada (Stothers and Metress, 1975). Sognnaes (1956, 1963), Brothwell (1963), and Clement (1963) have summarized the value of histological data from teeth in detecting carious lesions, developmental defects, chemical erosion, and dental mutilation.

Ericksen (1973) studied age-related internal remodeling of cortical bone in thin sections taken from the anterior femoral cortex of archeological recovered samples of Alaskan Eskimo, Southwestern Pueblo Indians, and Arikara Indians from South Dakota. She assessed internal remodeling by counting osteons, osteon fragments, and resorption spaces in three standardized microscopic fields. She found no differences among male populations but significant differences did occur among female groups. Ericksen proposes that extreme environmental stress upon the individual during pregnancy and lactation may account for the differences observed. Of course, the problem in age determination of the skeletons may also be a factor, but Ericksen has demonstrated the stimulating research possible with histological data.

Potential Use of Microscope

A number of other scholars have recently called attention to the potential of histological data in paleopathology research (Frost 1966; Putschar 1966; Blumberg and Kerley 1966; Armelagos 1967; Sandison 1968; and Stout and Teitelbaum 1976). Frost (1966: 132) noted that several skeletal disorders are pathognomonic with histological data including "vitamin D-resistant rickets [Frost 1964], osteomalacia, osteoporosis following injury, and Cushing's syndrome." Putschar (1966: 59) adds Paget's disease to the list with its histologically characteristic mosaic pattern. He appropriately noted that most other diseases which affect bone cannot be distinguished from skeletal evidence alone. For example, most of the candidates for pre-Columbia American syphilitic lesions cannot be distinguished confidently from those produced by other forms of periostitis. Despite these limitations, the Frost (1966) article indicates the potential for new information with intelligent interpretation of microanatomy. Frost noted that high osteon turnover can be expected in such disorders as "thyrotoxicosis, hyperparathyroidism, post-injury osteoporosis, and in the region of inflammatory lesions," (1966:140). Low osteon turnover usually accompanies "motor paralysis, Cushing's syndrome, hepatic cirrhosis, chronic alcoholism, diabetes mellitus, rheumatoid arthritis treated with salicylates, tertiary syphilis without periostitis, and chronic congestive heart failure," (Frost 1966:140). The ratio of resorption spaces to osteoid seams, cortical thickness, presence of fibrous bone in adult bone, and pattern of remodeling can all yield useful health information, especially when correlated with lines of arrested growth, dental defects or other radiographic or gross morphological information. Of course, overly simplistic models will produce dubious results, as demonstrated by the numerous diagnoses of syphilis in the literature. However, histological data can unquestionably add an important dimension to most studies and should be employed whenever appropriate.

Age Determination

In recent years, microscopic data have become important for the estimation of age at death. Of course, general age changes in bone development have been known for decades and summarized in numerous texts (Aegerter and Kirkpatrick 1969). Generally we know that three stages of bone development occur. The first occurs in the fetus and consists of the development from embryonic mesoderm of flexible cartilage in about the same shape and position of the later adult bone. This flexible skeleton is adequate in the fetus where structural support is not necessary and where flexibility is needed to enhance survival during the birth process.

During the first 18 months of life, primitive fiberbone replaces much of the cartilage, resulting in a more rigid skeleton than in the former stage. This bone does not have the strength of later adult bone, but it is sufficient for the young infant who is developing coordinated movements but does not yet need a durable skeleton for locomotion support.

As the need for support and movement increases, the fiberbone is slowly replaced with a stronger bone laid down in a stress-related pattern. During growth, increase in length is produced by activity at the epiphyseal plate while increase in width is accomplished by the periosteum. Throughout the growth process, shape is maintained through selective bone destruction (by osteoclasts) and production (by osteoblasts). (See Enlow 1963 for details.)

At maturity, epiphyseal and most periosteal bone growth terminates. However, internal cortical remodeling continues throughout the life of the individual. This remodeling functions to continually replace old bone with

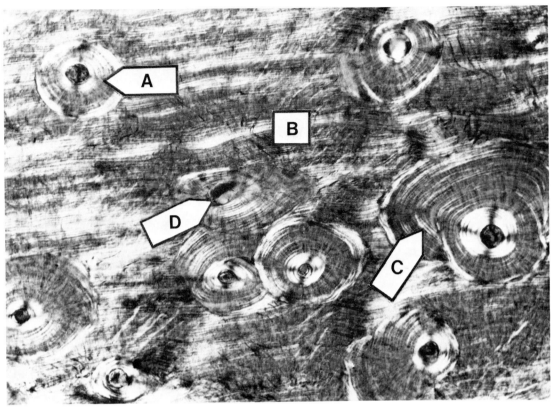

Fig. 11. Human adult cortical bone microstructure. (A) Secondary osteon; (B) Circumferential lamellar bone; (C) Osteon fragment; (D) Haversian canal.

new, structurally improved bone. Beginning early in life, osteoclasts cut canals through the original circumferential lamellar bone. These canals are then partially filled in by bone generated by osteoblasts. The entire resulting structure is called a secondary osteon and the remaining central canal is termed the Haversian canal (Fig 11). Some new osteons even cut through old osteons, leaving only fragments of the latter. The overall effect of this process is an increase with age in the number of osteons and osteon fragments at the expense of the original circumferential lamellar bone.

In 1965, Kerley published an aging method based upon the above process. Using a sample of 126 undecalcified sections of femora, tibiae, and fibulae taken from individuals of documented age at death, Kerley determined the effect of age on the amount of whole osteons, osteon fragments, non-Haversian canals, and circumferential lamellar bone. His

resulting aging method calls for counting the total number of osteons, osteon fragments, and non-Haversian canals, as well as the average percentage of circumferential lamellar bone in four circular visual fields placed on the periosteal margin of the cortex. The field size is that produced by a standard 10x objective with a wide field 10x eyepiece. The actual size is about 1.5 mm at the level of the section. Age at death can be estimated by using a chart or regression formulae. The equations present standard errors as low as 9.39 (femur), 6.69 (tibia) and 5.27 (fibula) years.

In 1969, Ahlqvist and Damsten pointed out: (1) that Kerley's reliance upon several structures for age assessment overly complicated the method while adding little accuracy; (2) that his use of circular visual fields necessitates specimen movement to distinguish structures on the borders of the field; and (3) that one of the visual fields he selected for examination falls directly upon the linea aspera, an area that demonstrates more nonage-related osteon variation than other areas. In their modified version of Kerley's method, Ahlqvist and Damsten consider only the total percentage of remodeled bone (osteons and osteon fragments) from four square fields placed just inside the outer surface of the bone. They spaced the fields around the circumference of the bone to fall between Kerley's fields and not on the linea aspera. Using a 100-square ruled ocular micrometer, inserted into the eyepiece so that one side (10 squares) of the grid measured one millimeter at the level of the section, they counted the number of squares more than half-filled with either osteons or osteon-fragments and represented the result as a percentage. Finally, by applying this method to 20 unstained, ground sections from midshafts of femora of known age at death, they developed a regression expressing the relation between age and the percentage of remodeled bone. Their linear regression formula contains a standard error of 6.71 years.

Using thin sections from the mandibles, femora, and tibiae of 59 cadavers of known age at death, Singh and Gunberg (1970) examined in two circular fields the total number of osteons, the average number of concentric lamellae per osteon, and the average diameter of the Haversian canals. From this data, they formulated regression equations with standard errors as low as 2.55 years (mandible).

Although the Singh and Gunberg method offers the lowest standard error of the three described, it is based upon a very restricted sample. The sample ranged in age from 40 to 80 years, with most individuals between ages 50 and 75. Thus the method is of limited importance in studying prehistoric samples in which most individuals are younger than age 50.

Of the remaining two methods, that of Ahlqvist and Damsten is probably the easier to employ because: (1) it does not require that osteons be distinguished from osteon fragments and (2) it is easier to count squares in the reticule than to count actual structures. However, the Kerley method is apparently much more accurate. Although the published standard errors are comparable, that of the Ahlqvist and Damsten method reflects a small sample of restricted age range. Recently,

Bouvier and the author (in press) applied both methods to a sample of Kerley's original femoral slides. The average error of the estimates made by the Kerley method was comparable to his published error. However, the error of the Ahlqvist and Damsten method increased to nearly 15 years when applied to the larger sample.

Although the Kerley method offers more accurate results, it should be used with caution. Some of the regression equations appear to be in error and the published field size of 1.25 mm is probably closer to 1.5 mm. Note also that a combination of 10x wide-field eyepiece and 10x objective can produce a field size from 1.2 to 2.0 mm, depending upon the structure of the microscope. Failure to allow for this variance can introduce an age estimate error as high as 33 percent. Until improved formulae on larger samples are available, it appears that the Kerley charts, based upon counts from about a 1.5 mm field size offer the superior results.

Age estimates from microscopic data also can be made using dental sections. In 1950, Gustafson published a method of determining age at death from seven features of dental microstructure: cemetum apposition, attrition, periodontosis, secondary dentin apposition, root resorption, transparency of the root, and closure of the root orifice. When considered together, these features produced age estimates containing a standard error of only 3.6 years. The standard curve was determined from a series of 41 teeth taken from individuals of known ages that ranged from 11 to 69 years.

Numerous modifications have been made on the Gustafson method since its formulation in 1950. Nalbandian (1959) and Nalbandian and Sognnaes (1960) found that experience was necessary to obtain reliable results and eventually duplicated Gustafson's findings. All investigators agree that Gustafson's method is accurate when employed by an experienced histologist with the proper sectioning equipment.

The methods documented above are those currently used to estimate age from microscopic data. However, other microscopic age changes have been documented. Jowsey (1960) documented that young individuals displayed a high frequency of new osteons and resorption spaces, obviously correlating with the extensive growth during that time in life. Young adults showed relatively low bone turnover, as evidenced by few forming osteons and resorption spaces. Older individuals displayed an increase in resorption activity with no increase in osteoblastic activity. This situation resulted in greater "porosity" and variation in mineral density. Jowsey also reported a higher incidence of plugged canals and filled lacunae during old age.

Sedlin et al. (1963) further documented Jowsey's resorption data by reporting that in 137 rib sections, the frequency of Howship's lacunae was highest in infancy, lowest in early-middle adult life and then higher in old age.

Using tetracycline labeling, Frost (1963) documented Jowsey's interpretation that osteoblastic activity slows with age. Frost found that in the rib, the time required to form a complete osteon from original resorption space was about 42 days at age 7.5 years but 79 days at age 43. He estimated that the formation requires 25 per cent more time in long bones.

In the same year, Villanueva et al. (1963) documented that new osteon formation correlated well with the resorption data of Sedlin et al. (1963). In their study of 139 rib sections, Villanueva et al. reported that the highest frequency of osteons with active osteoid seams occurred in infancy. The frequency then gradually decreased to a low at age 40 and then gradually increased into old age.

Currey (1964) studied nineteen femoral sections from individuals with ages documented from 23 to 89 years. In this small sample, Currey found that the amount of non-Haversian system bone (other than complete osteons) and number of Haversian canals (his indication of a complete osteon) increased with age. He found no age change in the size of the canal but explained the apparent contradiction of increasing number of new osteons with increasing non-osteon bone by noting that with age the osteons became smaller. He also noted that osteons became more circular and symmetrical with age.

In his study of 101 tibiae, aged 18 to 88 years, Ortner (1975) reported that in the outer cortex within the age limits of his sample: (1) the frequency of resorption spaces showed no age change; (2) forming osteons, newly formed osteons, and Haversian canal size in structurally complete osteons increased with age; and (3) osteons with high-density lamellae around their Haversian canals decreased with age. The variance in results between Ortner's study and others probably reflects the variability in structures examined and in their variable frequencies in different bones or different parts of the bone cortex. Ortner (in press) also has noted an age increase in the number and size of osteocyte lacunae per osteon.

All of these reports demonstrate both the need and potential for further research in pathological and normal age changes of bone microstructure. More detailed and better controlled studies are needed on larger samples from different populations. Greater knowledge of the variability among populations and within single populations is needed to intelligently assess data from prehistoric populations. Currently we apply microscopic aging methods to prehistoric bone on the assumption that the age changes are the same as those in recent populations. Future studies of the variability within recent populations should reveal if that application is valid or, if not, how the prehistoric data can be validated.

Slide Preparation

An important aspect of the histological examination of prehistoric tissue is the preparation of adequate thin sections. Good summaries are available for preparing stained sections of dessicated soft tissue (Allison and Gerszten 1975), decalcified stained bone sections (Andersen and Jorgensen 1960), microtome sections (Salomon and Haas, 1967) and staining (Frost 1959) of undecalcified bone, and ground sections of undecalcified bone (Moreland 1968; Ubelaker 1974). For most histological observations, especially those for age determination, I utilize undecalcified ground thin sections. Initially a 5- to 10-mm cross section is removed by using a sabre saw with a fine (32 teeth per inch) blade. From this initial section, a smaller (5-mm-thick) parallel-sided section is removed using an Ingram thin section cut-off saw (Model 103). Since most archeological specimens need to be thoroughly cleaned, they are immersed in Decal solution (available from Scientific Products) for about 50 minutes. This time allows the solution to dislodge and/or destroy foreign particles within the cortex without seriously damaging or decalcifying the bone itself. Throughout this period, the container of Decal is suspended in water within an Ultrasonic Cleaner, which helps the solution to penetrate the tissue as well as to remove the undesirable material. The section is then placed in water within the ultrasonic cleaner for an additional five minutes and then air-dried overnight.

Frequently the fragile condition of the important outer periosteal aspect of the cortex necessitates impregnation of the specimen. Accordingly, the specimen is placed overnight in a syrupy solution of equal parts of araldite (AY-105) and hardener (935-F) (both available from Chemical Coating and Engineering Co., Inc.) dissolved in toluene. Impregnation is most effective when accomplished under vacuum.

The impregnated specimen is dried in a 55° C oven overnight and then temporarily mounted on a glass slide with an acetone base cement. The free surface is then ground (Ingram Thin Section Grinder, Model 303) until it is flat. The specimen is then removed from the slide with acetone, and the previously ground surface is polished on a polishing wheel covered by polishing lap cloth. The cloth is coated with a three micron layer of diamond polishing compound, lubricated with A.B. polishing oil and A.B. mineral spirits.

Following this procedure the specimen is placed in acetone in the ultrasonic cleaner for one minute to remove the oil and diamond compound. The same araldite mixture described above without the toluene is then used to attach a glass slide to the polished surface of the specimen. A metal clamp should be employed to hold the slide and specimen together with even pressure. Prior to the actual attachment of the bone to the slide, all materials (araldite, hardener, bone, slide and clamp) should be heated to about 93° C on a hot plate. The specimen should be firmly attached in 20 minutes.

The specimen should then be reduced to a thickness of about 75 microns using the cut-off saw and grinder. Subsequently, the exposed surface must be polished and cleaned in the manner described earlier. After a cover-slip is attached with permount solution, the specimen is ready for analysis.

The entire procedure summarized above is presented in greater detail by Ubelaker (1974: 54–56) with some minor variation. Note that if the unprocessed specimen is well preserved and lacks the foreign particles of soil and fungus, then the immersion in Decal solution and impregnation would not be required.

Acknowledgments

I thank Stephanie Damadio and Donald Ortner for their careful reading and contributions to this manuscript and Eleanor Haley for her typing assistance.

THE OSTEOPATHOLOGY OF THE ROBINSON SITE SKELETONS*

DAN F. MORSE

The Robinson Site was excavated in the summer of 1963 by the University of Tennessee for the National Park Service. The excavations were in charge of Dan F. Morse. The site has been designated as 40Sm4, and is classified as "shell mound, Late Archaic." It is in Smith County, Tennessee, about 50 miles directly east-northeast of Nashville on the right side of the Cumberland River. Nine carbon 14 samples from this site were dated by the University of Michigan Memorial-Phoenix Project Laboratory. The period of occupation ranged from 1280 to 460 B.C. Sixty-two human burials were excavated. Most of these were badly disturbed and poorly preserved.

In 1966, the most obvious pathology, consisting of portions of 13 burials recorded by Dan F. Morse, were shipped from the University of Tennessee to Peoria.** These were examined and described by Dan Morse, M.D., of Peoria; A. J. Novotny, M.D., orthopedic surgeon, Peoria; and Don Brothwell of the British Museum of Natural History, London. The following is their description of these specimens. With the exception of one burial, No. 55, only the pathological portions were available for examination. The skeletons of the Robinson Site are in the permanent collection of the McClung Museum, Department of Anthropology, University of Tennessee, Knoxville.

***

**Examination of the Robinson Site skeletons was through the courtesy of Dr. Alfred K. Guthe, Head of the Department of Archaeology, University of Tennessee.

BURIAL NUMBER: 4   Male   Age 26
DESCRIPTION:
  HUMERUS: The distal half of the right humerous shows a deformity consisting of widening and anterior-posterior flattening with slight anterior angulation. The articular surface of the lateral condyle is partially destroyed—which could limit extension to approximately 135 degrees. The medial epicondyle is irregular, as is the entire lower half of the humerus.
  ULNA: The distal seven-eighths of the right ulna is thickened. There are two small areas of irregularity on the right radius, indicative of inflammatory changes.
DIAGNOSIS: Inflammatory changes of right arm are probably due to trauma.
DISABILITY: Pain in arm and some limitation of motion. Process was probably active at time of death and thus may have been a contributory cause.
PLATE NUMBER: 34,A

***

*From unpublished Ph.D. Thesis, University of Michigan, 1967, by Don F. Morse, now with the Arkansas Archaeological Survey, Jonesboro, Arkansas.

BURIAL NUMBER: 5   Female   Age 29
DESCRIPTION:
    RIGHT FEMUR: This is a healed fracture at the proximal third in the region of the neck
                      and trochanter, with a 40-degree anterior angulation. Much callus forma-
                      tion is present, indicating the possibility of some infection after the trauma,
                      which was probably a compound fracture.
    RIGHT PATELLA: Normal.
    RIGHT TIBIA: This is also a fracture of the upper third with overriding and shortening.
                      There is a 30-degree varus angulation. The medial tibial condyle shows
                      lipping, probably due to mechanical strain. There is a bony bridge union
                      between tibia and fibula at fracture site.
DIAGNOSIS: Fractures of upper right femur and upper right tibia.
DISABILITY: This individual had a pronounced limp and was handicapped as far as
                      running and stooping. The right leg must have been two to three inches
                      shorter than the left. There is a moderately severe arthritis of the right
                      knee which may have restricted movement.
PLATE NUMBER: 33,H and 34,B

BURIAL NUMBER: 9   Female   Age 30
DESCRIPTION: The third right upper molar is impacted and nonerupted. The upper right
                      canine is partially erupted but has been deflected laterally as there is no
                      space between the lateral incisor and the medial premolar.
DIAGNOSIS: Impacted molar and crowded canine in maxilla.
DISABILITY: Probably none. May have had pain.
PLATE NUMBER: 34,C

BURIAL NUMBER: 11   Female   Age 30
DESCRIPTION: The great toe of the left foot shows severe arthritis of the interphalangeal
                      joint with lipping. The middle phalanx of another toe has a small exostosis
                      on dorsal surface.
DIAGNOSIS: Traumatic arthritis.
DISABILITY: Probably none. May have had some pain.
PLATE NUMBER: 33,C

BURIAL NUMBER: 22   Male   Age 32
DESCRIPTION: Only a few vertebral fragments are available for study. These show pro-
                      nounced osteoarthritis, lipping and irregularity of the intervertebral sur-
                      face of two thoracic and three or four lumbar vertebrae.
DIAGNOSIS: Severe osteoarthritis.
DISABILITY: Probably severe back pain.

BURIAL NUMBER: 24   Female   Age 35
DESCRIPTION: Minor enlargement, indicating healed fracture of the shafts, of the left
                      ulna and radius at the junction of the middle and distal thirds.

| DIAGNOSIS: | Fractures of left ulna and radius. |
| DISABILITY: | Good results with no disability after healing. |

BURIAL NUMBER:	25 Sex not determined Age 13
DESCRIPTION:	Teeth show moderate wear. Both lower third molars are unerupted and impacted. The skeletal age is only 13, but the general opinion is that the teeth would probably have remained impacted.
DIAGNOSIS:	Impacted mandibular wisdom teeth.
DISABILITY:	Probably none.
PLATE NUMBER:	34,C

BURIAL NUMBER:	30 Female Age 26
DESCRIPTION:	Healed fracture of the middle third of the left humerus with slight angulation.
DIAGNOSIS:	Fracture of left humerus.
DISABILITY:	None after healing, good results.

BURIAL NUMBER:	31 Female 50+
DESCRIPTION:	
VERTEBRAE:	Fragments of two cervical vertebrae show moderate osteoarthritic changes with lipping and irregularity of joint surfaces.
SKULL:	On the left parietal in the region of the pterion, there are changes on the external and internal surface. Externally, there is an elliptical area measuring approximately 25 by 15 mm. of raised and pitted bone. Internally, the major impression for the middle meningeal artery has an eroded and enlarged appearance, indicative of a pathological process.
DIAGNOSIS:	Indefinite. The process started internally and was eroding through the bone. Possibilities are brain abscess or infected thrombus.
DISABILITY:	Possible acute illness with death.
PLATE NUMBER:	33,F and 34,D

BURIAL NUMBER:	43 Male Age 40
DESCRIPTION:	The frontal sinus region displays severe bilateral sinusitis. At the angle made by the left upper orbital margin and temporal line is a large "sinus" opening, and from this lesion the infection appears to have spread up the scalp over the frontal and along the upper part of the parietals (displayed by some vault thickening and pitting of the external surface). The right glenoid fossa shows osteoarthritic changes. It is possible that the region of inflammatory discharge at the left frontal angle may originally have been the seat of penetrating injury into the sinus. The clavicle shaft fragment shows minor irregularity and enlargement, possibly the result of an osteitis.
DIAGNOSIS:	Infection of the scalp caused by trauma involving frontal sinuses.
DISABILITY:	Active at time of death and probably the cause.
PLATE NUMBER:	33,A

Burial Number: 52   Female   Age 50
Description: On the internal surface of the posterior-inferior portion of the body of both mandibular rami is a small, follicular cyst-like indentation. The size of the left cyst is about 1.0 cm. and the right 0.3 cm. These are not symmetrically located, as the cyst on the right is a little more anterior. Five small follicular indentations can be seen on the left and two follicles on the right.
Diagnosis: Follicular bone cysts.
Disability: None.
Plate Number: 33,B and 34,D

Burial Number: 55   Female   Age 45
Description:
    Vertebrae: Fragments of at least six vertebrae are available for study. Four are cervical, one of which is the atlas. All of these show severe osteoporosis with irregularity of most surfaces. One articular facet of the atlas and several other articular facet fragments show severe osteoarthritic changes. The two vertebrae identified as thoracic are also osteoporotic; one of these is severely flattened and wedge-shaped.
    Skull: The skull is available for study. The bones of the skull show no evidence of osteoporosis. The skull shows a smooth rounded hole into each antrum to admit the root of the second molar. The wall of the right maxillary sinus is thickened, the result of the chronic sinusitis possibly spreading through molar root penetration or apical infection.
Diagnosis: This is a puzzle. Localized vertebral osteoporosis is rare. This may be Cushing's disease.
Disability: Severe, probably leading to death. Wedging or compression of thoracic vertebrae is due to osteoporosis. A terminal injury to the spinal cord is the probable cause of death.
Plate Number: 33,D and 34,C

Burial Number: 58   Female   Age 22
Description:
    Right Maxilla: There is a small hole in the right antrum to admit the root of the molar. The wall of the maxillary sinus appears to be normal.
    Mandible: On the external aspect of the left ramus is much evidence of a thin layer of subperiostial new bone and this extends to the linguinal aspect of the coronoid process.
    Left Maxilla: The left side of the maxilla also shows areas of subperiosteal new bone and this inflammatory reaction extends back onto the molar. The same process has produced an osteitis in the region of the glenoid fossa and the external auditory meatus.
Diagnosis: Active inflammation at time of death of right side of face involving the soft tissues, with bone reaction.
Disability: Severe facial infection probably resulting in death.
Plate Number: 33,G

APPENDIX 2

THE CRABLE SITE

Dan F. Morse

The Crable Site, named after a previous owner, Mr. Norman Crable, is situated on a bluff near the Illinois River and Anderson Lake in the extreme southeastern corner of Fulton County, Illinois. A spring is present on the eastern-facing bluff slope at one edge of the main site concentration. The well-defined bluff rises 160 feet above the surrounding bottomlands. The bluff surface extends about 10,000 feet from north to south and varies in width from 200 to 1,500 feet. The northern end of the bluff contains the Fiedler Site and Mounds (Morse, Schoenbeck and Morse, 1953). The southern end, now a part of the Roger Briney farm, contains thirteen of the Rose Mounds (Baker, Griffin, et al., 1941).

The Crable Site itself is considered to occupy a 75-acre area on the bluff top and eastern slope. The greatest concentration of village debris is found in a 10-acre "mound field," designated by the University of Chicago as F^{v}891. About in the center of this concentration is a large "temple mound" (F°898). About 1,000 feet to the north is the "mound ridge." On this ridge were four mounds, one of which was excavated by Edgar McDonald and his father in 1932 (McDonald 1950). The other three mounds were excavated by the University of Chicago in the summer of 1933 (Smith 1951). Five cemeteries as identified by Edgar McDonald were located on ridges adjacent to the mound field.

The Crable Site has attracted sporadic occupations from terminal glacial times to the present. Evidence of Paleo-Indian, Archaic, Hopewell and Late Woodland camps have been found, besides the enormous quantity of Middle Mississippian debris indicating the probability of several successive Mississippian occupations.

Archaeological excavations, which included the Crable Site, were conducted in Fulton County, Illinois, by the University of Chicago during the period of 1929 to 1933 under the directorship of Dr. Fay-Cooper Cole (Cole and Deuel 1937). Those directly connected with this investigation at Crable include: Dr. Hale G. Smith, who wrote his M.A. thesis in anthropology at the University of Chicago on this site (Smith 1951); Dr. Robert J. Braidwood, who was the surveyor and draftsman; Dr. Thorne Deuel, who directed the field party in 1933; Dr. J. D. Jennings, who supervised the excavations; and Dr. Georg Neumann, who was the osteologist. The only other scientific excavation at the site was a four-day visit in 1964 under the general field direction of Dr. Georg Neumann and the direct supervision of Dan F. Morse. This was an Indiana University-National Science Foundation Summer Institute in Anthropology excavation. A number of local collectors have visited the site for the past hundred years or so (*History of Fulton County, Illinois,* 1879). Most notable of the recent excavators were Roy Clayton, H. Edlin, Glen McGirr and Edgar and Charles McDonald. Most recently a large surface collection has been accumulated by Dr. Dan Morse. In addition to the complete destruction of the cemeteries in the early 1930's, the site is eroding away at an alarming rate; and lately random digging by various individuals has decreased the value for further scientific investigation.

In July, 1967, the Allis-Chalmers Company leased the entire bluff (1,200 acres) from the owner, Roger Briney, for use as a proving ground for heavy machinery. The Illinois State Museum has negotiated with the equipment company so that archaeological investigations can be completed before the destruction of the various Indian sites. These sites include all of Crable and portions of the Fiedler village and the Rose Mounds. It is hoped that a great deal of valuable information will be accumulated.

The Village

Village debris is scattered over the entire 75 acres with several areas of concentration, the principal area being the 10-acre "mound field." Most of the information concerning the village site is derived from materials collected on the surface. Excavations in the village have been sparse, consisting of a few garbage and food storage pits. No house remains have been investigated. The University of Chicago placed two test pits in the southwest portion of the mound field (Smith 1951), and Indiana University excavated a 160-square-foot area to the west.

Artifacts recovered give evidence of a year-round occupation, with important economic basis on agriculture. A large variety of pottery styles include bottles, bowls, deep plates and jars. Most pots were undecorated or covered with cordmarked impressions caused by hitting with a cord-wrapped paddle. Some were painted with a red film and many were incised with simple geometric designs. Bowls sometimes had an animal effigy head appendage added to the lip. Pottery was also used to make perforated discs and elbow-shaped pipes. The discs may be gaming devices. Perforated deer toes used in the pin-and-cup games and stone discoidals for rolling on the ground almost certainly were gaming items.

Stone projectile points are small in size and triangular in shape. About 3 percent of these are notched near the base. Some projectile points are made of deer antler. Chert knives, scrapers, gravers and drills are also relatively common items found on the site surface. Other utilitarian stone artifacts include ungrooved axes, hoes, abraders and hammers. Two significant chert artifacts, a micro-drill and portions of long knives are similar to items found in an early period at Cahokia near St. Louis, Missouri. Copper is rare, but artifacts of shell (beads, gorgets, spoons, hoes), bone (awls, fishhooks, scrapers, chisels, scarifier sets), and antler (handles and flakers) are common.

During the 1964 excavation by the Indiana University-National Science Foundation Summer Institute in Anthropology, a large test pit was placed in the village. This is in addition to the investigation of the platform mound which will be described later. This test pit measured 13.5 by 17.0 feet and was located approximately 250 feet southwest of the platform mound. A good deal of Middle Mississippian debris was obtained. This included Middle Mississippian pottery sherds, triangular projectile points, sandstone abraders, and scrapers, and various worked flint and bone tools. In one feature within this pit was a 7.0-by-8.0-foot oval area of debris, burned logs, and portions of two adult human skeletons. The fragmentary log sections measured 2.5 to 3.0 inches in diameter and were oriented and distributed discontinuously within the feature. Skeleton 1 was represented by two lower legs *in situ* which indicated it originally had been oriented extended on its back with the skull pointing southwest. Shell beads were scattered among the foot bones, in a single 2-foot-long line beneath the feet, and in two short parallel rows on a nearby potsherd. These beads included convex-sided 1.0-by-1.5-cm.-in-diameter long beads; 1.7-by-0.9-cm.-long disc beads; and a "spiro knuckletype" or double bead measuring 0.7 cm. in diameter and 1.4 cm. long. The second skeleton was represented by these *in situ* bones: a pelvis, a sacrum, and a few vertebrae. These indicated a skeleton oriented on its back with the skull pointing westward. It is obvious that more investigative excavations are advisable in order for better understanding and interpretation.

Carbon 14 Dates

Three dates run by the University of Michigan Radiocarbon Laboratory are available (Crane and Griffin 1959). These have recently been corrected and are as follows:

		Range
M-550	590±100 B.P. (A.D. 1360)	A.D./1260-1460
M-553	620±100 B.P. (A.D. 1330)	A.D./1230-1430
M-554	530±100 B.P. (A.D. 1420)	A.D./1320-1520

(B.P. is "before the present." The B.P. values are subtracted from A.D. 1950 according to a decision made by the Fifth Radiocarbon Dating Conference to obtain a Christian-era calendar date.)

Sample M-550 was collected by Dr. James B. Griffin from a post mold a few feet inside the freshly cultivated field near the south gate, and Dr. Dan Morse forwarded the charcoal he collected for samples M-553 and M-554 from a refuse pit along with all associated artifacts to Dr. Griffin.

The Platform Mound (F°898)

This mound has been estimated as being originally 30 to 40 feet high in 1879 (probably an exaggeration by the author of *History of Fulton County*); 10 or 12 feet high and 60 feet in diameter, according to McDonald (1950); and 15 feet high and truncated in 1933, according to Smith (1951). In 1964, the Indiana University excavation reported that the mound was conical in outward appearance, 6 feet high, and measuring between 100 and 150 feet on a side. The mound as well as the general flat area immediately to the southwest, which may be a plaza, is relatively sterile of artifacts.

An exploratory trench was dug into the mound measuring 44.8 feet long and 7.0 feet wide. The cross section revealed the following construction phases: Of the total of seven post molds intruding into the natural subsoil, four appeared to be part of a large circular structure (possibly 47 feet in diameter) which may have existed before the actual mound was constructed. These four measured 9 inches in diameter, extended to depths ranging from 14 to 26 inches beneath the surface of the original top soil, and were spaced 4 to 5 feet apart. Although no indication of a packed floor was observed, it was thought that this was a ceremonial structure, probably of pre-mound vintage or at least associated with the initial construction of a platform mound. Though not packed hard, the surface of the 2.5-foot-thick primary strata was quite horizontal. It was made up of a mottled series of sandy loam and clay lenses. A thin charcoal and sand streak was just beneath the top of this strata and may be a part of the floor of a structure.

The next stratum added was a 1.8-foot-thick layer of gray clay. Superimposed on the surface of this layer are no less than five packed floors. Each floor is represented by a packed 2-cm.-thick charcoal layer with intervening thin layers, from bottom to top, as follows: a 0.25-cm.-thick brown clay and sand, a 0.25-cm.-thick brown clay and sand, a 1-cm.-thick mottled brown clay, and a 0.50-cm.-thick gray layer.

Superimposed over the fifth charcoal layer is the basal remnant of a third major mound stratum which has been mainly destroyed by cultivation and random mound pitting. This final layer is made up of light brown clay.

Because of the almost total absence of village debris in the mound, it is apparent that the mound fill was not obtained from the surrounding village and, furthermore, the occupants of the village must have respected the mound area since it was not littered with refuse.

Mound Ridge

Four mounds were located on a ridge north of the main village concentration. The McDonalds excavated a part of one of the mounds, and the other three were investigated by the University of Chicago. The McDonalds worked on the southern portion of the mound designated as F°895. They found a great deal of refuse material, plus a "number of bundle or disturbed burials" near the top and some extended burials near the base. No artifacts were associated with the former; of the latter, one had a cache of projectile points and another had a vessel with four lugs.

The University of Chicago excavated the other three mounds. Mound F°892 produced two extended burials with red-ocher-stained bones. No artifacts were associated. Mound F°893, only partially excavated, produced fragments of a skeleton and a Maples Mills (Late Woodland) firepit. Mound F°894 was completely excavated and found to have been constructed over 11 extended and flexed burials whose graves intruded into a Maples Mills camp. Associations were meager, consisting of a rectangular shell gorget, two bone needles, one triangular projectile point and miscellaneous debris which could have been accidentally included in the grave fill.

The Cemeteries

A total of four cemeteries have been excavated at the Crable Site by McGirr and the McDonalds. Two were on the bluff ridges, south of the spring. The other two were on ridges near "Mound Ridge," to the northeast.

McDonald (1959) reported that possibly as many as two to three hundred skeletons were present in the largest Crable cemetery investigated. The smallest cemetery, after having been dug by McGirr and the McDonalds, still contained 28 undisturbed skeletons at the time of the University of Chicago investigation.

Descriptions of the artifacts recovered from the four cemeteries are found in Smith (1951), Morse (1960) and McDonald (1950). In contrast to the general village debris, the cemeteries produced some quite exotic artifacts. Bone pins included one with a human effigy carved on the base. Shell gorgets are incised discs, some decorated with elaborate geometric designs. Included are a stepped or "cloud motif," the cross motif, and spider and eagle effigies. Shell rattles and copper-covered wooden ear spools also occur. A 10-inch chert mace and five chert swords ranging from 9⅝ to 15½ inches in length are probably the most spectacular items present.

Exotic pottery includes a water bottle with a short straight neck and a series of negative-painted crosses and dots on the body; an effigy bowl with an inverted rim, representing an owl lying on its back; a beaker with a handle which represents a clenched human fist; a compound vessel consisting of two bowls joined by a central bar; a blank-faced effigy bottle; a variety of beakers and incised bowls; and both deep and shallow plates.

All in all, the general picture is an earlier complex than those reported by Smith (1951) from the village excavations. Similarities to earlier Southern Cult sites such as Etowah are striking. Adequate notes on grave lots and locations were not kept by the collectors of the exotic artifacts and no one is very sure of the significant context of the artifacts collected.

The McDonald collection, which includes 120 pottery vessels, 1,100 projectile points, 4 ceremonial swords, 2 spider-engraved gorgets, 12 fishhooks, and numerous other items such as beads, knives, celts, scrapers, etc., was purchased by Mr. William Rutherford for the Forest Park Foundation, Peoria, Illinois. The purpose of this acquisition was to keep this part of the Crable collection intact for future study. The Foundation has loaned this collection to the Lakeview Center Museum of Peoria, Illinois.

The Dr. Dan Morse Crable collection consists of over 5,000 chert arrows, knives and scrapers. There are 21 large pots and eight miniature or "toy" pots which were obtained from the original McGirr collection. In addition there are literally hundreds of stone, shell and bone tools and ornaments, plus many bushels of pottery sherds.

Some of the McGirr material is at Dickson Mounds Museum. There are a few specimens at the Museum of the American Indian, Heye Foundation, New York; but the bulk of the collection is owned by Mrs. Gene B. Whiting, Montrose, Alabama.

Interpretation

It is very likely that all of the skeletal material at the Dickson Mounds Museum, labeled "Crable," was from the cemeteries. Whenever the McDonalds or Mr. McGirr found something they considered abnormal, they presented that portion of the skeleton to Don Dickson. It is certain that these specimens belonged to Indians of the Mississippian culture, but the exact time within the Mississippian period cannot now be determined, principally because no records were kept of the location of the specimens or artifact association.

There are four questions one might ask about the Crable Site. However, none of these questions can be answered satisfactorily, with only the knowledge available.* It is hoped that future exhaustive scientific investigation will be conducted on this important Indian site so that more accurate information can be obtained concerning the following:

(1) Where did the inhabitants of Crable come from?

(2) How long was Crable occupied by the Mississippian people?

(3) What kind of life did they have?

(4) And finally—what happened to them?

At the present time there is no evidence that there is any connection between the Late Woodland Camp found at "Mound Ridge," and the Mississippian culture located in the village, the cemeteries and the mounds. Mississippian did not develop from Late Woodland at Crable, nor did the Mississippian and

---

*At the present time (summer, 1969) the Department of Anthropology, University of Illinois—Chicago Circle, is engaged in extensive field excavations at the Crable Site under the direction of Dr. Robert L. Hall.

Woodland mix together there. Hence, Crable was settled by Indians coming in from another area, sometime during the Mississippian period.

Since there is almost a total absence of "Early" or "Old Village" Mississippian material (thin polished black and brown pottery called "Powell Plain" and "Ramey Incised," rolled rims on the jars, multiple notched small arrows, micro-drills, etc.), this settlement must have occurred essentially after "Old Village," possibly around A.D. 1200-1300. Since there is no apparent stratification of culture material in the village excavations, one could infer, as Smith did, that Crable was not inhabited by a few people for a long period of time but many people for a short time. It could be further inferred that this was during the Late Phase because of the numerous Oneota-like traits found both in the cemeteries and the village. The same pottery traits have been found on Oneota sites in Wisconsin and Iowa. These include a profusion of globular-shaped small jars, with rims oriented outward and incised rectilinear decorations such as "trees," "chevrons," lines and punctates (Griffin 1960: 809-865). On the other hand, many of the artifacts from the cemeteries and some from the village are more likely to be identified with the Middle Phase of the Mississippian culture. All village site excavations have been conducted in the concentrated "Mound Field." It is possible that investigation in adjoining fields may demonstrate the presence of an earlier component. We know that occupation of the site ceased before historic times in Fulton County as no iron, glass, or other historic artifacts have been found dating to the initial historic period.

In a *History of Fulton County*, written in 1879, the following quote is taken from Chapter XI, entitled ARCHAEOLOGY: "One of the most outstanding points of interest in the county is located on Sections 31 and 32 in Kerton Township. Here, on the surface of a high bluff, is a field on the land of a Mr. Fisher, known as a 'Mound Field,' perhaps 25 acres, that may properly be called a city of the dead. . . . And here are the remains of not less than one hundred and fifty thousand human beings buried literally by the cord."

Obviously this is an exaggeration, but such a statement would indicate that there were a great number of human burials. Add to this the fact that literally thousands of artifacts have been recovered from the village site, mostly from the surface, and we arrive at the impression that the population at Crable must have been considerable. This would mean some dependence on agriculture. How much cannot be determined with our present knowledge. There has been no pollen or seed analysis and no evidence of garden plots in the vicinity. On the other hand, Dr. Paul Parmalee, Zoologist, Illinois State Museum, has examined material from several refuse pits and identified an abundance of mammal, bird and fish bones in addition to many species of freshwater mussel shells. Almost all mammals, birds and fish known to have existed in this area, except bison, have been found.

From the illustrations in this book, one is aware that the people of Crable suffered from many diseases and injuries. There were numerous instances of arthritis, osteomyelitis and fractures. The large collection of Crable skulls at the Dickson Mounds Museum demonstrates the existence of a variety of dental abnormalities and pathology. So far, we have no reason to believe that a stockade surrounded the village. The location on a high bluff with a view overlooking the surrounding countryside would suggest a favorable situation for defense if needed. The presence of the temple (platform) mound and the profusion of grave goods indicates that religion and ceremony played an important part in the lives of the inhabitants.

Smith (1951) had the Crable Site inhabited by the Illinois Indians, more specifically the Peoria, because: (1) the Peoria ". . . were the only ethnic group in the area," and (2) ". . . there is no sharp break between the Spoon River aspect of the Mississippian and the Oneota." Griffin (1960) also appears to see the Peoria developing out of Spoon River. Griffith further states that the very late Mississippian material around Starved Rock, Illinois, is remains of the Kaskaskia. The Kaskaskia were another Indian tribe belonging to the Illinois Federation. All the carbon dates at Crable, so far, center around A.D. 1400. It is possible that there was a time period when the area in Fulton County was uninhabited and that there may have been a space of one to two hundred years between the last of the Crable and the first of the Peoria. Historical accounts certainly do not indicate that the number of Peoria Indians in early historic times were anywhere near the dense population that we believe to have existed in late Crable time.

In a personal communication, Dr. Georg Neumann, Chief of the Department of Physical Anthropology, Indiana University, after examination of some of the Crable skeletal material at Dickson Mounds, stated that from the viewpoint of the physical anthropologist, it is very unlikely that Crable contained the immediate ancestors of the Peoria. If this is true, then there must be another reason to explain what happened to them. There has never been a very satisfactory explanation to account for the disappearance of the Mississippian Indians in many of the sites thoughout the Midwest. One inference is that there may have been a severe drought or spell of cold weather lasting for several years, causing a succession of crop failures and forcing movement to other areas. Another possibility is the introduction of diseases which could have wiped out most of the population and caused the few survivors to flee to the south or west and to have lost their identity when they joined other tribes. Warfare also could have accounted for the end of the Mississippian culture, but there is no archaeological or historical evidence for this.

In summary, the Mississippian Indians at Crable did not develop from the Late Woodland people that preceded them but moved into the area sometime after A.D. 1200 and stayed on until late prehistoric times. The latter part of their stay was characterized by a large population. Their economy depended on farming, hunting and probably food gathering. Ceremony and religion played a major role in their lives. What happened to them is a puzzle.

THE ARCHAEOLOGY OF DICKSON MOUNDS

During the years 1966 to 1968, archaeologists from the Illinois State Museum have been engaged in scientifically excavating an area at Dickson Mounds in order to remove all skeletons and archaeological material that otherwise would be destroyed by the construction of a new museum building. The study of all collected artifacts, skeletons, maps, photographs, drawings, measurements and recordings will literally require years before the complete story of Dickson Mounds will be known. So far, it is clearly apparent that Indians occupied the Dickson Site for a very long time, perhaps as long as five centuries: from Late Woodland through almost all of the Mississippian Period. This fact makes Dickson Mounds one of the most valuable archaeological sites in the Midwest.

For more of the story, we must wait for future publications. Now the archaeology of Dickson Mounds can best be understood by extracts from previously published articles. One of these, by Don Dickson himself, deals with the mounds before the latest excavations. Another, by Dr. Joseph Caldwell, formerly Curator of Archaeology at the Illinois State Museum, tells something about the recent discoveries.

DICKSON MOUNDS*

DON F. DICKSON

Dickson Mounds, comprising 63.25 acres, was acquired by the State of Illinois in 1945. It is easily reached from Routes 97 and 78 and is about five miles from both Havana and Lewistown. The Mounds are situated three-quarters of a mile from the Spoon River, which joins the Illinois River near Havana. This beautiful valley has been made famous by Illinois' great poet, Edgar Lee Masters, who frequently referred to it in his writings.

MOUND EXHIBIT IS UNIQUE

The mound exhibit is unique in many respects. It consists of a prehistoric Indian cemetery-mound in which burials and offerings have been left as they were placed many centuries ago. More than 200 graves can be seen in the 30-by-60-foot excavation. This site has been known as a prehistoric burial mound for more than a century. It was in the Dickson family for four generations.

At an early period, when pioneers were clearing the hill for farming and a home site, many burials were found. In subsequent farming and excavating for buildings and through natural soil erosion, burials and artifacts were encountered. This has continued down through the years.

BODIES IN ORIGINAL POSITIONS

The plan of uncovering the burials in their original positions in the soil was started in 1927. At first temporary structures protected the excavation. Later a permanent building was constructed.

---

*Taken from *Dickson Mounds* by Don F. Dickson, an informational folder published originally by the Illinois State Department of Conservation and reprinted in 1967 by the Illinois State Museum with minor revisions by Joseph R. Caldwell.

Under State ownership the site is being preserved as one of Illinois' two most spectacular archaeological centers, the other being Cahokia Mounds State Park near East St. Louis.

The mound, which is on the Illinois River bluffline, gives the visitor a magnificent view of thousands of acres of river floodplain. No location could have been more attractive to the American Indian. An abundant food supply was assured by access to the river, lakes and marshes of the Illinois Valley. Protection was to be found in the bordering hills. And perhaps the Indians in this spot were moved, no less than we, by its natural beauty.

THE FIRST AMERICANS

From the time the Europeans landed in America and contacted its inhabitants, man has been studying the first Americans. That interest has never subsided. Because the Indians lacked any form of writing, historians and scientists are unable to obtain the complete story without resorting to archaeology and its many allied sciences.

The Indian probably entered America more than 15,000 years ago. With the development of tree-ring chronology and radiocarbon dating, the dates of the various aboriginal cultures are being established.

INDIANS SUPPOSEDLY CAME FROM ASIA

The accepted theory is that the first Americans came from Asia and probably used the Bering Strait region as a point of entry. By gradually spreading southward they eventually peopled North and South America.

All American Indians belong physically to the great Mongoloid division of mankind, but there are many differences among tribes. Variations undoubtedly developed due to geographical differences, climate and food. It is thought all American Indians had a common origin.

There are more than 10,000 mounds and village sites scattered over Illinois, the largest number, more than 1000, being in Fulton County. All mounds, however, are not for burial purposes.

MADE VARIOUS TYPES OF MOUNDS

Mound building in North America began about 1000 B.C. Most of the earliest mounds

were for burial, but the Indians later constructed enormous geometric earthworks whose purpose can only be conjectured. Some later Indians made effigy mounds in the shape of turtles, mammals and birds over one or more bodies.

Mound building was being carried on at about the time the first plants began to be cultivated. With the growing of corn, pumpkins, squash and beans, the people gradually achieved a more settled kind of life. Some founded towns and religious centers, often with temples and public structures erected on flat-topped earthen mounds and sometimes protected by a palisaded wall.

THE DICKSON MOUND

The mound measures approximately 550 feet from one point of the crescent around to the other. The depression is between the arms of the crescent, and in this area we find the loess soil from which the mound was built. This wind-blown soil is an excellent natural preservative of bones and was the easiest to handle.

BURIALS SHOW ARTISTIC DEVELOPMENT

Archaeological investigations reveal an artistic development and a high degree of spiritual achievement. There are many evidences of elaborate ceremonial customs. Many possessions were buried with the remains.

In some instances many beautiful artifacts are associated with a burial, but with some burials there are few, if any, possessions. Much of the material buried with the dead has perished.

Frequently many rare and beautiful artifacts are found in the graves of tiny children, even premature babes. Some of the rarest and most artistic pieces are in graves of those too young to have used them.

Perhaps we can learn through archaeology of some of the finest and most beautiful qualities of man.

MUCH INTERESTING PATHOLOGY

The life expectancy of the prehistoric Indian was comparatively short, due largely perhaps to a high death rate in infancy. Accidents and infections were numerous, and arthritis and bone deficiency diseases were not uncommon.

In addition to the skeletons in the excavation there are on display many exhibits of bone and dental material from other sites. These show some of the diseases, fractures, deformities and anomalous developments in bones and also in teeth.

Many authorities in pathology believe the Europeans brought to the Indians such diseases as smallpox, measles, scarlet fever, diphtheria, malaria, yellow fever and typhoid.

MANY DISEASES ARE FOUND

On display are examples of prehistoric arthritis, osteomyelitis, tumors and many fractures and abnormalities. The average teeth were good but by no means perfect. There are examples of most of the dental diseases and anomalies encountered today.

Pyorrhea was present. Examples of dental caries, wear, supernumerary or displaced teeth, congenital absence of one or more teeth, impactions and abscesses affecting both the teeth and surrounding bone are also on display.

ONLY SMALL SEGMENT EXCAVATED

The present work is but a small portion of the entire mound. It is interesting to see over 200 skeletons in so small a space and to try to reconstruct the story represented. The mound contains skeletons from top to base and from one side to the other.

THE TOMB IS NOT SILENT

The tomb is not silent, however, on some points. In it you can see not only that which is of value to the archaeologist but also a beautiful story of a brave people who lived here long before Columbus discovered America.

These "first Americans" made articles with such thought for the practical that in their pottery you will find a design similar to almost every type in use today.

In some respects it is the most remarkable exhibit of its kind in the world, and there have been visitors from every country to see it. Archaeologists and scientists from many of the larger institutions of the country have found it of great interest in their study of the aboriginal inhabitants of this continent.

VILLAGE SITE PRESERVED

The story of these early Indians would be incomplete without a study of their village. In 1928, two prehistoric house sites were located on the hill west of the mound. Nearby, natural springs provided an ample water supply.

In 1959, it was discovered that another group of prehistoric buildings extended to the south. An excavation was started in this area under the supervision of the Illinois State Museum. A continuation of this work will provide a story of this prehistoric village.

Evidence of seven buildings has been uncovered so far. The traces of these were detected at approximately eighteen inches below the present ground level. The floors were originally at this depth, and there seems to have been very little erosion or building up of the soil in this area since the time the Indians lived here. All that remains after the passage of time is evidence of postholes and wall trenches which once held supporting wall timbers. Sometimes, charred remains of roof beams or other logs are also found. Some imprints, fragments of wattled walls, and clay-plastered and grass- or reed-thatched roofs have been preserved.

Some of these buildings were probably used as dwellings, others as public structures. One was circular in shape and another was a very large rectangular building which was probably covered with earth. At some time it caught fire and many of the timbers, including part of the roof, were found preserved as charcoal.

The most unusual building found to date was in the shape of a Greek cross. Compass readings showed it positioned only nine degrees off the present magnetic North. A radiocarbon date for this building is A.D. 1300.

FOOD PRESERVED AS CHARCOAL

Each of the houses had one or more hearths. On the floors of some of them and in storage pits nearby is evidence of the kinds of food the Indians ate.

Bones of many small animals have been found in and around the village area. Available to these prehistoric people were such animals as the black bear, raccoon, badger, skunk, mink, fox, wolf, woodchuck, squirrel, beaver, muskrat, elk, deer, and bison. There has also been evidence of fish, birds, turtles, and mussels.

The Indians who occupied this village were definitely agriculturists, producing corn, pumpkins, squash, beans, and gourds. Also available to them were acorns, hickory nuts, pecans, hazelnuts, black walnuts, butternuts, wild rice, maple sugar, wild cherries, gooseberries, blackberries, plums, and grapes.

Many fragments of pottery have been found as well as flint and stone tools, mussel shell hoes, and some large, flat mortars, usually of sandstone. The latter were used for grinding foods such as corn and nuts.

AGE OF THE VILLAGE

A number of radiocarbon determinations

suggest that the buildings south of the mound belong to the period A.D. 950-1200. The burials in the mound are later, belonging to A.D. 1200-1400. The homes of these people were scattered along the bluff on which the mound is situated.

In archaeological parlance the occupations represented at this site are known as "Mississipian" and they show the effects of strong influences from the south, especially from the Cahokia region near present-day East St. Louis.

Several shells originating in the Gulf of Mexico are associated with burials. Some of these are cut for use as bowls or dippers; others, with a groove or a perforation at the small end, were ornaments to be suspended from the neck.

NEW DISCOVERIES AT DICKSON MOUNDS*

JOSEPH R. CALDWELL**

The plan to build a new and much larger museum at Dickson Mounds required investigation of archaeological remains outside the present museum building to prevent their being destroyed by the new construction. These excavations, conducted this summer, have provided unexpected insights into the nature of Dickson Mounds. More surprisingly, they tell of events which took place there before the mound was built.

About A.D. 700-900 during a period called "Late Woodland," long before the building of the mound, a village occupied this section of the Illinois River bluff. Here, during the last summer's excavation, was found part of a wooden palisade which probably surrounded

the settlement. So far no houses have been found, but some storage and cooking pits, chipped stone artifacts, and fragments of thin, grit-tempered pottery have been uncovered. Some of the pottery is plain surfaced (Sepo Plain), some is cord-marked (Sepo Cord-marked), and some is partly smoothed after cord-marking (Sepo Smoothed-over Cord-marked). Vessel rims usually show extra decoration, ticks or notches on the inside or the outside, and sometimes one or two horizontal impressions of a single cord, again either on the inside or the outside of the rim.

The same kind of pottery has been found on the floors of houses in a later village close-by, the Eveland Site below the Illinois River

*Reprinted from *The Living Museum,* Vol. XXIX, No. 6, Oct. 1967, Springfield, Illinois State Museum, pp. 139-142.
**Dr. Caldwell, formerly Head Curator of Anthropology at the Illinois State Museum, is now Professor in the Department of Anthropology, University of Georgia.

bluff. Intermingled with this older pottery at the Eveland Site is a new exotic ware exactly like that used during the 12th and 13th centuries at the great town of Cahokia near the present East St. Louis, Illinois. This later ware is tempered with shell instead of grit. It is sometimes polished (Powell Polished Plain) and sometimes carries, in addition, attractive incised running decorations on the shoulders of the vessels (Ramey Incised). There are also some less carefully made vessels (Eveland Incised and Eveland Plain) which look like local imitations of the foreign ware. The exotic pottery probably originated in the Cahokia area, but it is also widespread in the prairie areas north and northwest of Cahokia. In a number of instances it is associated with varieties of Late Woodland pottery, as is found at the Eveland Site.

Until this past summer there was much speculation as to whether or not Eveland might be a settlement of invaders from the Cahokia area who adopted, as pioneers often do, some of the indigenous traits of the region while maintaining their essential identity. Now this seems less likely, for the discovery of the little village on the bluff tells us that there was a Late Woodland population in the area of the present park with a pottery-making tradition that continued throughout the occupation of the newer village down below. Moreover, it has also been learned that the inhabitants of the Eveland Site buried their dead in the ruins of the old village on the bluff, some burials even cutting into the place where the palisade once stood. At the present writing more than thirty burials of these people have been found. The skeletons are semi-flexed, i.e., the knees are drawn up toward the abdomen, as is often characteristic of Late Woodland burials. The hypothesis of Cahokia invaders does not fit the newly discovered facts nearly as well as an hypothesis that a resident Late Woodland population somehow became "acculturated" under the influence of Cahokian ideas and customs This kind of phenomenon is one that is often seen today when developing countries come under the influence of technologically more advanced nations. Just how this happened at Dickson Mounds is not known, but to recognize the problem is the first step in solving it.

What military, political, religious or economic factors were at work is not known. What is known, however, are some of the effects of these unknown factors. From these something of the nature of the influences may someday be inferred.

These efforts were tremendous. At just about the same time that the Cahokian pottery appeared at Eveland, erection of a series of large temple mounds was started along the Illinois River from present day Beardstown to Peoria, each seven to ten miles apart, each evidently serving the cluster of villages and hamlets within walking distance of it. Each cluster was thus a community (which incidentally provides the archaeologist with a social dimension of study) very much like the so-called "towns" of the historic Creek and Cherokee Indians which included all the inhabitants of a locality using the same "town house," which in older times was on the temple mound. Probably, as in the case of the Creeks and Cherokee, these communities strung along the Illinois River considered themselves part of a larger community and sometimes acted in concert.

Another great change which seems to have taken place at this time, or at least now becomes visible, was a cultural orientation to the prairie, perhaps as a result of increased interaction with those people north and west of Cahokia who had also fallen under Cahokian influence. The elaborate constructions at the Eveland Site include what appears to be a large earth lodge and a domestic dwelling following the exact pattern of the Wichita grass house. Two bison scapular hoes have been found in the Illinois Valley, one of these at Eveland. Here, too, were found numerous chipped stone "end scrapers," a well-known prairie-plains tool.

The Eveland Site was abandoned about A.D. 1200. Shortly afterward, the Illinois bluff was again occupied by a much larger village. The inhabitants of this village had what archaeologists call a Mississippian culture (Spoon River focus) which closely resembles that of Cahokia of about A.D. 1300-1400. Both, in turn, have a close cultural resemblance to many large towns and villages along the Mississippi, the Ohio and the Cumberland rivers. It is as if the old Cahokian sphere of influence or interaction with the northwest prairie areas had become relatively less important while a new sphere of interaction grew up in the general region of the Ohio and the central Mississippi Valley.

There are some indications in the last village of Dickson bluff of a cultural transition from Eveland. The new village could have been a lineal descendant of the Eveland community. At the time of this last habitation the burial mound was begun and, perhaps significantly, it was built directly over the old Eveland cemetery.

Understanding of the burial mound has also changed considerably as a result of the recent investigations. The loessic soil of which the mound was built does not easily disclose the disturbed earth by which grave pits can be recognized. It was formerly believed that there were no grave pits, that the mound had grown as a result of bodies being laid successively on the surface of the ground with earth heaped over them. It has since been determined that the bodies were put in dug graves and that on at least two occasions the height of the mound was increased by adding great layers of additional earth.

The new excavations have also presented some puzzles. There are parts of the mound where burials are heavily concentrated, other parts where there are no burials at all. There are parts of the mound where burials are aligned in one way, other parts where they are aligned differently. There are parts of the mound where particular kinds of grave offerings are present and other parts where other kinds of offerings appear. Is this mound composed of family or clan plots? Will it eventually be possible to infer something about the social organization of the town from the distinctions made in the burial of the dead? The new excavations have revealed much that was not known. Above all, it is obvious that at Dickson Mounds the story is just beginning to unfold.

A BRIEF REVIEW IN OSTEOLOGY

ROBERT C. DAILEY AND GINA M. COMER*

Introduction

This appendix will consider aspects of human osteology not found in the text but which are by way of review supplemental to the body of knowledge contained therein. To fully determine pathologies and abnormalities in skeletons, it is advantageous to be familiar with the normal characteristics of the skeleton. Only a general representation of the normal human skeleton (as in Figure 12) will be presented here with referrals to easily available literature for further details. It should be stressed that this appendix serve as a guide to standard references with no claims to be definitive.

Identification and Description

The 206 bones in the normal human skeleton are classified by shape into four categories: (1) long—possessing a shaft and two extremities (see Figure 14); (2) short—a miniature long bone; (3) flat—possessing extended surfaces for muscle attachments; (4) irregular—odd/distinctive shapes. Separation into these categories initially will aid in the identification of individual bones. Such relationships may be as in Figure 13. The next determination, adult vs. subadult status, is best estimated from factors involving eruption of dentition and consequent wear, epiphyseal closure and the relative development in length of the long growth bones. See Bass's laboratory manual (1973) for aid in this estimation or consult an expert osteologist. Then, placement of an individual bone in proper cranial or postcranial position is best achieved when envisioned in standard anatomical position.

* Department of Anthropology, Florida State University.

Bass (1973) is of particular value in determining right from left in paired bones and provides cursory attention to the description of all bones found in the human skeleton. A good standard medical anatomy text is also of great instruction in the detailed description of each individual bone and its relationship in articulation with other bones, see Goss et al., *Gray's Anatomy* (1966). For unique illustrations (in particular roentgenographic), consult Pansky and House (1971) and Becker, Wilson and Gehweiler (1971).

Some of the most diagnostic features in the identification of an individual be it normal or pathologic in character can be obtained from the dentition. For the best discussion of dentition, the reader should consult Anderson's (1962) manual in addition to Bass (1973).

It is most often the case that a skeleton to be analyzed is in fragmentary condition. Expertise in the identification of bone fragments is a requisite to further study of any abnormalities present. Such knowledge can be gained through experience and serious study. When in doubt confirmation by an expert osteologist is highly recommended.

Discontinuous Morphology (Nonmetrical Variations)

Anthroposcopic studies, formerly a peripheral concern of anthropometry, can be quite informative in individual and population studies. Human skeletal plasticity as manifested in nonmetrical variants or discontinuous morphological traits can be accounted for with the utmost facility and expediency— a simple scoring of the feature as regards its presence or absence. The recording of such anomalies is of particular significance in the

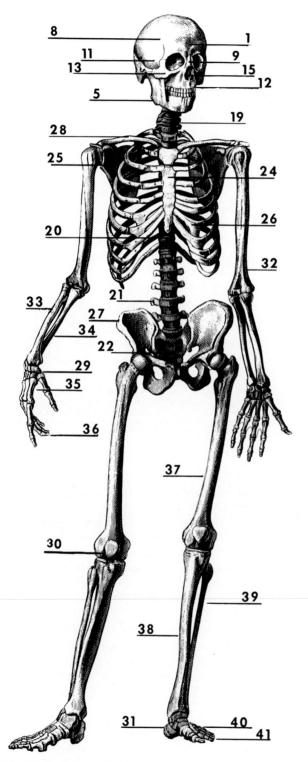

Fig. 12. The human skeleton.

THE BONES OF THE NORMAL HUMAN SKELETON

CRANIAL BONES (29)

	SINGLE (7)	PAIRED (22)
F L A T	1.Frontal 2.Occipital* 3.Vomer*	8.Parietal 9.Nasal 10.Lacrimal*
I R R E G U L A R	4.Sphenoid* 5.Mandible 6.Ethmoid* 7.Hyoid*	11.Temporal 12.Maxilla 13.Zygomatic 14.Palate* 15.Inferior Nasal Concha 16.Malleus* 17.Incus* 18.Stapes*

POST CRANIAL BONES (177)

	SINGLE (27)	PAIRED (150)

I R R E G U L A R	19.Cervical
	  vertebrae(7)
	20.Thoracic
	  vertebrae(12)
	21.Lumbar
	  vertebrae(5)
	22.Sacrum
	23.Coccyx*	

F L A T	24.Sternum	25.Scapula 26.Ribs(24) 27.Innominate
S H O R T		28.Clavicle 29.Carpus(16) 30.Patella 31.Tarsus(14)
L O N G		32.Humerus 33.Radius 34.Ulna 35.Metacarpus(10) 36.Phalanges(28) 37.Femur 38.Tibia 39.Fibula 40.Metatarsus(10) 41.Phalanges(28)

*not clearly visible in figure

assessment of a skeletal population. Again, an understanding of the normal adult human skeleton and its anomalies is essential to a comprehensive knowledge of evidence for pathologic conditions. Some of the more common variants are metopic suture, perorate sternum, os inca, accessory ossicles and septal aperture. Nonmetrical variations have received most notable attention by Brothwell (1963), Berry (1968) on cranial aspects and Anderson (1962, 1968) particularly on post-cranial aspects.

Estimations of Race, Stature, Age and Sex

It is important for students of paleopathology to know, wherever possible, the racial affiliation, sex, age and to some extent the stature of the skeletons under examination. With this information differential rates of mortality and disease frequency may be determined and compared. Racial affinities of recent skeletons are difficult to determine because of the degree of hybridization which is characteristic of modern populations. Consequently, very little has been published which clearly and unambiguously permits the easy identification of skeletons with respect to race. Krogman (1962) outlined some of the better known criteria which can be used in the identification of Causcasoid and Negroid skeletons. Burial context is also of considerable importance in this assessment. Indeed it is often the case that the method of burial and associated artifacts will help confirm an identification which can be only hazarded at best. Anderson's manual *The Human Skeleton* (1962) provides a useful outline of burial practices and criteria to consider in identifying American Indian populations.

Stature estimation is considerably precise. Several methods have been developed, one by Dupertius and Hadden (1951) and the other, which is more widely used, by Trotter and Gleser (1958) involving factors correcting for racial affinity. The latter procedure is thoroughly presented in Bass's manual *Human Osteology* (1971). Other manuals which may be consulted for these and other methods of stature estimation are Swedlund and Wade's *Laboratory Methods in Physical Anthropology*

by Swedlund and Wade (1972) and *Introduction to Physical Anthropology, Laboratory Manual* by Kelso and Ewing (1962).

There are a number of criteria which may be used to estimate the age of skeletons. These include eruption of the dentition, changes in the face of the pubic symphysis and epiphyseal union. Eruption of the dentition is quite easily determined in the normal adult cranium, though x-ray examination may be necessary where the third molar is found to be absent. Two methods of assessing age based on changes in the face of the pubic symphysis are available and recommended. That of Todd is included in the manual by Bass (1973), and the other devised by McKern and Stewart is included in the manuals by Kelso and Ewing (1962) and Swedlund and Wade (1972).

Estimation of the sex of a human skeleton may be assessed using a number of criteria. Male skeletons usually possess heavy muscle markings and more pronounced protuberances and tuberosities than female skeletons, but it is a mistake to assume that sexual dimorphism (intraspecific differences between the sexes) is always reliable. Indeed, one has to know the limits of a particular breeding population before assessment involving grossness/gracility can be relied upon, and even at best the discrimination is tenuous. Again as in the case of age, the pelvic (innominate) bones are the most critical for the determination of sex and considerable reliance can be placed on estimations if these bones are intact. Bass's manual contains an excellent discussion of the differences between the male and female pelvis. Additional discussion of sexing can also be found in Kelso and Ewing (1962) and Swedlund and Wade (1972).

Retrieval of Skeletal Material

Careful excavation and collection of skeletons is a must in order to achieve accuracy and avoid long hours of difficult reassembly in the laboratory. Recently this has been emphasized in homicide investigations, whenever buried bodies are involved (Morse et al. 1976). Frequently the paleopathologist has no control over how the bones are collected and also, too frequently, receives them incom-

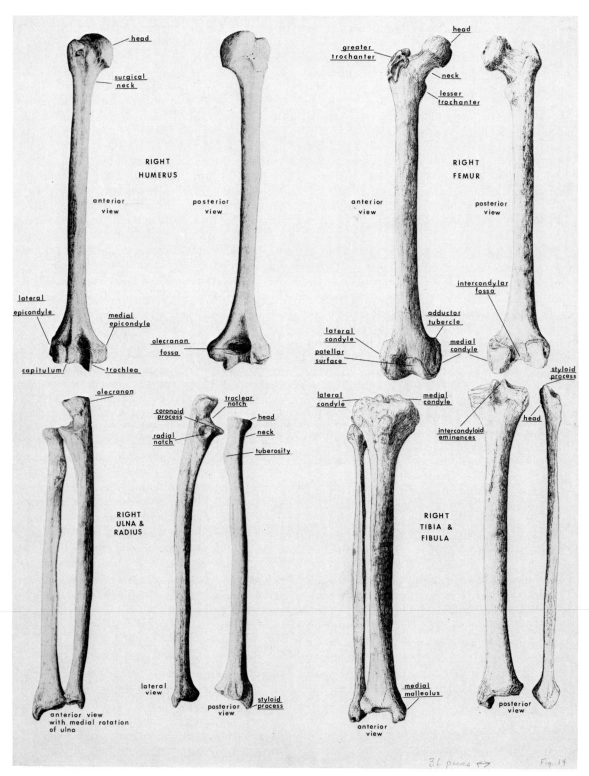

Fig. 13. Long Bones.

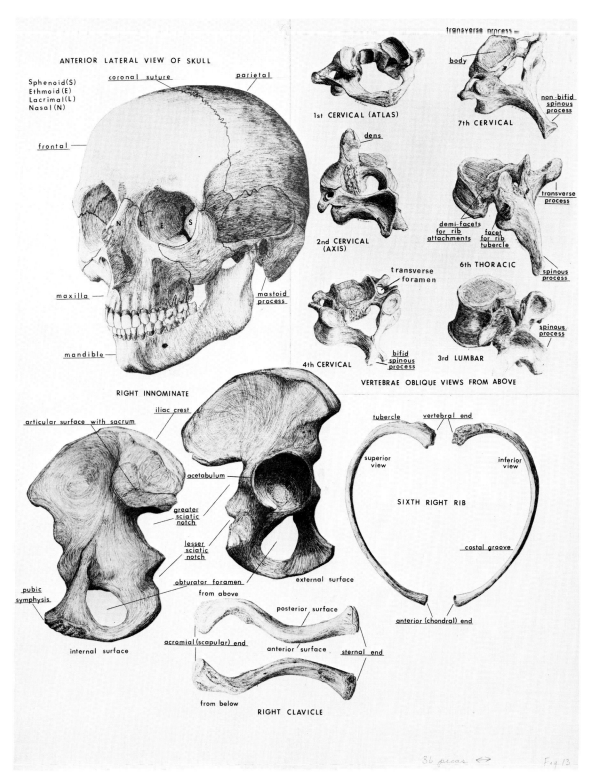

Fig. 14. Some bones of the skeleton.

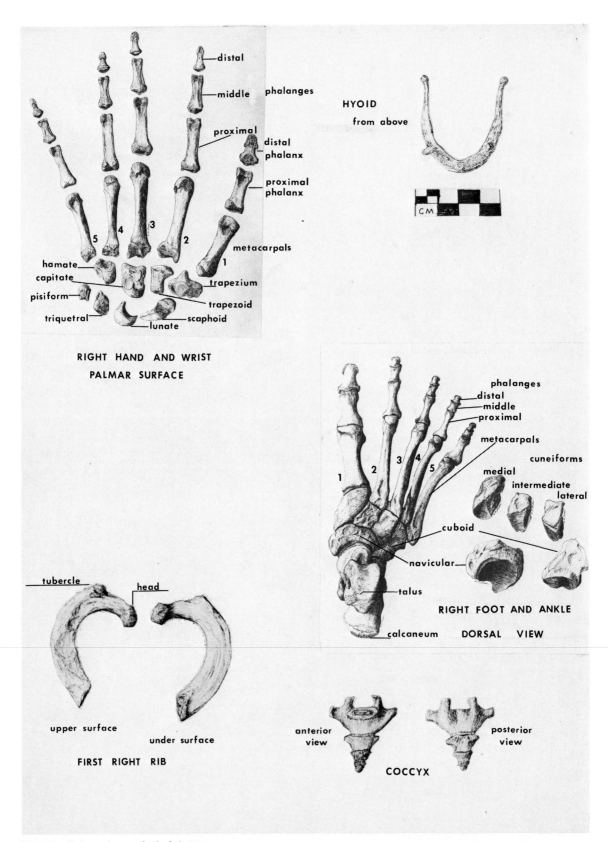

RIGHT HAND AND WRIST
PALMAR SURFACE

distal
middle — phalanges
proximal
distal phalanx
proximal phalanx
metacarpals
hamate
capitate
pisiform
triquetral
trapezium
trapezoid
scaphoid
lunate

HYOID
from above

CM

phalanges
distal
middle
proximal
metacarpals
cuneiforms
medial
intermediate
lateral
cuboid
navicular
talus
calcaneum

RIGHT FOOT AND ANKLE
DORSAL VIEW

tubercle
head
upper surface
under surface

FIRST RIGHT RIB

anterior view
posterior view

COCCYX

Fig. 15. Commonly overlooked bones.

plctc, damaged and with entire bones missing. If possible the paleopathologist should see the bones *in situ* while they are being excavated and should be given some supervisory power in their removal. Proper packaging, labeling and transportation to the laboratory should be of concern to the specialist who intends to analyze skeletal material. An inventory of the bones should be made at the time they are being removed from the ground. If any are missing, this should be recorded after a careful search has been completed. Some of the smaller bones are extremely fragile and will decay rapidly; but even when present, they may be overlooked as their coloring will be similar to the soil. The packaging should be done in a manner which makes the examination in the laboratory more rapid. A separate container for each hand and foot labeled right and left is highly recommended. Those small bones most commonly overlooked—hyoid, coccyx, carpals, and tarsals—are presented in Figure 15.

Forensic Considerations

No two skeletons are exactly alike. There is always some variation manifest. In forensic investigations, these variations, whether congenital or acquired, have been used to identify or eliminate a missing suspect who may be the skeletonized victim. Antemortem medical records and x-rays should be obtained for this purpose. A valuable procedure in such cases is to compare the dental records of the suspects with the skeleton. Care must be taken not to rule out a certain suspect until all possibilties and characteristics have been considered. In modern practice, an x-ray is usually taken before dental work is begun. However, changes can occur between the time the records were made and the time of death. Additionally, one must consider that a dentist's records are often completed only to the extent felt necessary in the treatment of the patient. The dentist may not list the presence or absence of such anomalies as Carabelli's cusp, etc. We are aware of one instance in which the presence of a supernumerary tooth was not recorded. Again, many mistakes have occurred in antemortem records, such as right from left, upper from lower, etc. It is advisable to consult a forensic odontologist in the confirmation of a judgement. Figure 16 is a suggested form for the recording of dentition of a skeleton. It is equally adaptable to both archaeological and modern specimens and is a combination of the universal (Luntz and Luntz, 1973) and Brothwell (1963) systems.

DENTAL ANALYSIS

DEPT. OF ANTHROPOLOGY   FLORIDA STATE UNIVERSITY

LOCATION (SITE #)_____ BURIAL # OR NAME_____
SEX_____ AGE_____ RACE_____
DESCRIPTION OF SPECIMEN: _____
_____
_____

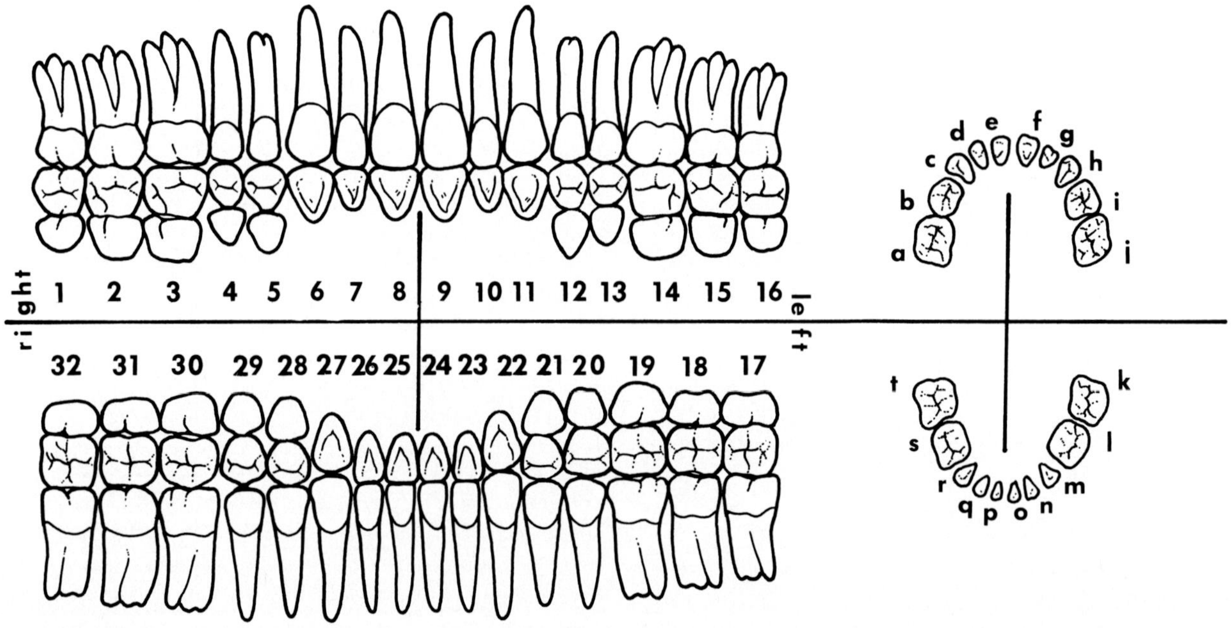

LEGEND:

X   tooth lost postmortem (socket present)   //// area missing
/   tooth lost antemortem (socket filled)   T   tarter
ʊ   tooth not yet erupted   0   occlusion
C   cavity (size & location -indicate by outline) Ps   prosthesis
A   abcess (draw in)
F   filling (describe in notes,indicate by shading)
Ab   abnormalities (describe in notes)
Py   other pathology (notes)

ATTRITION: DESCRIPTION:
1. None to slight (enamel only)   _____
2. Enamel plus dentine (slight)   _____
3. Enamel plus dentine (heavy)   _____
4. Pulp exposure (with or without   _____
      formation secondary dentine)   _____
                                              _____
PERIDONTAL DISEASE (resorption of bone):   _____
1. Less than 2mm. from neck   _____
2. and 3. in between   _____
4. Exposure of entire root   _____

USE OTHER SIDE FOR ADDITIONAL NOTES

Fig. 16. Form for recording teeth.

TABLE 5

CULTURES REPRESENTED BY PATHOLOGY DESCRIBED IN TEXT

SITES	PALEO-INDIAN (10,000+ B.C.)	ARCHAIC Early (8,000 B.C.)	ARCHAIC Late	WOODLAND Early (1,000 B.C.)	WOODLAND Middle	WOODLAND Late	MISSISSIPPIAN Early (A.D. 1000)	MISSISSIPPIAN Middle	MISSISSIPPIAN Late	HISTORIC (To A.D. 1600)
INDIAN KNOLL			x							
MODOC		x	x							
ROBINSON			x							
MORSE			x			x				
KLUNK			x		x	x				
DOGTOWN					x					
BLUE CREEK					x					
STEUBEN					x	x				
WEAVER					x	x				
FREDERICK					x	x				
RIVIERE AUX VASE						x				
DICK'S MOUND						x				
NUTWOOD						x				
BEAR CREEK						x				
INDIAN MOUND PARK						x				
PETER'S MOUND						x				
CAHOKIA						x	x	x		
THOMPSON							x			
ROSE							x	x		
SCHILD							x	x		
VANDEVENTER								x		
BECKSTEAD								x		
EMMONS								x		
MOUNDSVILLE								x		
BERRY								x		
DICKSON						x	x	x	x	
CRABLE								x	x	
KANE								x	x	
FISHER									x	
BRADLEY									x	
CHUCALISSA									x	x
BANKS									x	x

x — Culture represented by pathology described in text

Note: *Red Ocher* is a Late Archaic
      Bluff and *Weaver* are Late Woodland
      Hopewell is Middle Woodland

REFERENCES CITED

Ackernect, E. H.
1955. Paleopathology. In *Anthropology Today*, A. L. Kroeber (Ed.). University of Chicago Press, Chicago, pp. 120–126.

Adis-Castro, Elias and Georg K. Neumann
1948. The Incidence of Ear Exostosis in the Hopewell People of the Illinois Valley. *The Proceedings of Indiana Academy of Science*. Vol. 57, pp. 33–36. Bloomington, Indiana.

Aegerter, Ernest and John A. Kirkpatrick, Jr.
1969. *Orthopedic Diseases*. W. B. Saunders Company, Philadelphia. Third Edition.

Agassiz, L.
1833–43. Recherches Sur les Poissons Fossiles, Neuchatel.

Ahlqvist, J. and O. Damsten
1969. A Modification of Kerley's Method for the Microscopic Determination of Age in Human Bone. *Journal of Forensic Sciences*. Vol. 14, No. 2, pp. 205–212.

Alexandersen, V.
1967. The Pathology of the Jaws and Temperomandibular Joint. In *Diseases in Antiquity*, Brothwell and Sandison (Ed.). Charles C Thomas, Springfield, Illinois. pp. 551–595.

Allison, M. J. and E. Gerszten
1975. *Paleopathology in Peruvian Mummies*. Virginia Commonwealth University, Richmond.

Allison, Marvin J., Enrique Gerszten, Raul Sotil and Alejandro Pezzia
1976. Primary Generalized Hyperostosis in Ancient Peru. *Medical College of Virginia Quarterly*, Vol. 12, No. 2, pp. 49–51.

Allison, Marvin J., Daniel Mendoza and Alejandro Pezzia
1973. Documentation of a Case of Tuberculosis in Pre-Columbian America. *American Review of Respiratory Disease*, Vol. 107, pp. 985–991.

Allison, Marvin J., Alejandro Pezzia, Enrique Gerszten, Ronald F. Giffler, and Daniel Mendoza
1974. Aspiration Pneumonia Due to Teeth 950 A.D. and 1973 A.D. *Southern Medical Journal*, Vol. 67, No. 4, pp. 479–483.

Allison, Marvin J., Alejandro Pezzia, Enrique Gerszten and Daniel Mendoza
1974. A case of Carrion's Disease Associated with Human Sacrifice from the Huari Culture of Southern Peru. *American Journal of Physical Anthropology*, Vol. 41, No. 2, pp. 295–300.

Allison, Marvin J., Alejandro Pezzia, Ichiro Hasegawa, and Enrique Gerszten
1974. A Case of Hookworm Infestation in a Precolumbian American, *American Journal of Physical Anthropology*, Vol. 41, No. 1, pp. 103–106.

Andersen, Helge and J. Balslev Jorgensen
1960. Decalcification and Staining of Archaeological Bones, with Histochemical Interpretation of Metachromasia. *Stain Technology*, Vol. 35, No. 2, pp. 91–96.

Anderson, J. E.
1962. *The Human Skeleton. A Manual for the Archaeologist*. National Museum of Canada, Ottawa.

Angel, J. Lawrence
1967. Porotic Hyperostosis or Osteoporosis Symmetrica. In *Diseases in Antiquity*. Brothwell and Sandison (Ed.). Charles C Thomas, Springfield, Illinois. pp. 378–389.

Armelagos, George J.
1967. *Future Work in Paleopathology*, Museum of Northern Arizona, Technical Series No. 7, pp. 1–8. Flagstaff.

Ascenzi, Antonio
1970. Microscopy and Prehistoric Bone. In *Science in Archaeology*. Don Brothwell and Eric Higgs (Eds.), Praeger Publishers, New York, pp. 526–538.

Baker, F. C., J. B. Griffin, R. G. Morgan, G. K. Neumann and J. L. B. Taylor
1941. Contributions to the Archaeology of the Illinois River Valley. *Transactions of the American Philosophical Society*, Philadelphia. Vol. 32, Pt. 1, pp. 22–28.

Bass, William M.
1971. *Human Osteology. A Laboratory and Field Manual*. Missouri Archaeological Society, Columbia, Missouri.

Becker, R. Frederick, James W. Wilson and John A. Gehweiler
1971. *The Anatomical Basic of Medical Practice*. The Williams and Wilkins Co., Baltimore, Md.

Benfer, Robert A. and Thomas W. McKern
1966. The Correlation of Bone Robusticity with the Perforation of the Coronoid-Olecranon Septum in the Humerus of Man. *American Journal of Physical Anthropology*, Vol. 24, No. 2, pp. 247–252.

Bennett, Kenneth A.
1965. The Etiology and Genetics of Wormian Bones. *American Journal of Physical Anthropology*. Vol. 23, No. 3, pp. 255–260.
1967. Craniostenosis: A Review of the Etiology and a Report of New Cases. *American Journal of Physical Anthropology*. Vol. 27, No. 1, pp. 1–9.

Benninghoran, C. D. and E. R. Miller
1942. Coccidiodal Infection in Bone. *Radiology*. Vol. 38, p. 663.

Berg, Ed.
1972. Paleopathology: Bone Lesions in Ancient Peoples. *Clinical Orthopaedics*, No. 82, pp. 263–267.

Black, Glen A.
1967. Angel Site. *Indiana Historical Society*. Indianapolis. pp. 549–551.

Bloom, William L., John L. Hollenbach and James A. Morgan
1965. *Medical Radiographic Technique*. Charles C Thomas, Springfield, Ill. pp. 34–37, 105–107.

Blumberg, Joe M. and Ellis R. Kerley
1966. A Critical Consideration of Roentgenology and Microscopy in Palaeopathology. pp. 150–170. In *Human Palaeopathology*. Saul Jarcho (Ed.). Yale University Press, New Haven.

Bosworth, D. M. and J. Levine
1949. Tuberculosis of the Spine. *J Bone Joint Surgery* (Amer), Vol. 31, p. 267.

Bouvier, Marianne and Douglas H. Ubelaker
In press. A Comparison of Two Methods for the Microscopic Determination of Age at Death. Submitted for publication *American Journal of Physical Anthropology*.

Bowers, Warner F.
1966. Pathological and Functional Changes Found in Pre-Captain Cook Contact Polynesian Burials from the Sand Dunes at Mokapu, Oahu, Hawaii. *International Surgery*, Vol. 43, No. 2, pp. 206–217.

Broesike, G.
1882. Ueber die feinere Structur des Normalen Knochengewebes. *Archiv Mikrosk. Anat.*, Vol. 21, pp. 695–765.

Brooks, Shelagh T. and Jerome Melbye
1967. Skeletal Lesions Suggestive of Pre-Columbian Multiple Myeloma. Technical Series No. 7. *Miscellaneous Papers in Paleopathology:* 1, William D. Wade (Ed.). Museum of Northern Arizona, Flagstaff. pp. 23–29.

Brothwell, Don R.
1963. *Digging up Bones*. British Museum of Natural History, London.
1963. The Macroscopic Dental Pathology of some Earlier Human Populations. In *Dental Anthropology*. Don Brothwell (Ed.), Pergamon Press. London, pp. 271–288.

Brothwell, Don R. and H. Graham Carr
1962. The Dental Health of the Etruscans. *British Dental Journal*, Vol. 113, pp. 207–210.

Brothwell, Don R. and A. T. Sandison
1967. *Diseases in Antiquity*. Charles C Thomas, Springfield, Illinois.

Browthwell, Don R. and Vilhelm Moller-Christensen
1963. Medico-Historical Aspects of Mutation. *Danish Medical Bulletin*, Vol. 1, No. 1, pp. 21–26.

Brothwell, D. R., A. T. Sandison and P. H. K. Gray
1969. Human Biological Observations on a Guanche Mummy with Anthracosis. *American Journal of Physical Anthropology*, Vol. 30, No. 3, pp. 333–347.

Brown, James A.
1961. The Zimmerman Site. *Illinois State Museum Reports of Investigations*, No. 9, Springfield, Illinois.

Burke, R. M.
1955. *An Historical Chronology of Tuberculosis*. Charles C Thomas, Springfield, Illinois.

Calabro, John J.
1965. Chronic Arthritis. *Arthritis and Related Disorders*, American Physical Therapy Association, New York. pp. 35–42.

Caldwell, Joseph R.
1967. New Discoveries at Dickson Mounds. *The Living Museum*, Vol. XXIX, pp. 139–142. Illinois State Museum, Springfield, Ill.

Carter, Mary E. (Ed.)
1963. Radiological Aspects of Rheumatoid Arthritis *International Congress Series 61*. Excerpa Medica Foundation, Amsterdam.

Clement, A. J.
1963. Variations in the Microstructure and Biochemistry of Human Teeth. In *Dental Anthropology*. Don Brothwell (Ed.), Pergamon Press, London, pp. 245–269.

Cole, Fay-Cooper and Thorne Deuel
1937. *Rediscovering Illinois*. University of Chicago Press, Chicago.

Cole, H. N., J. C. Harkin, B. S. Kraus and A. R. Moritz
1955. Pre-Columbian Osseus Syphilis. A. M. A. *Archives of Dermatology*, Vol. 71, pp. 231–238.

Collins, D.H.
1966. *Pathology of Bone*. Butterworth, London.

Cooper, Norman S.
1965. Arthritis and the Rheumatic Diseases—Pathologic Considerations. *Arthritis and Related Disorders*. American Physical Therapy Association, New York. pp. 11–20.

Crane, H. R. and J. B. Griffin
1959. University of Michigan Radiocarbon Dates IV. *American Journal of Science Radiocarbon Supplement*, Vol. 1, pp. 181–186.

Cruxent, J. M. and I. Rouse
1958. An Archaeological Chronology of Venezuela. *Social Science Monographs VI*, Pan American Union, Washington, D.C. Vols. 1, and 2.

Currey, J. D.
1964. Some Effects of Aging in Human Haversian Systems. *Journal of Anatomy*, London, Vol. 98, No. 1, pp. 69–75.

Curtis, C. S. and E. G. Loomis
1941. Bone Tuberculosis in Northern Newfoundland. *J Bone Joint Surgery* (Amer), Vol. 23. pp. 812–813.

Dahlberg, Albert A.
1949. The Dentition of the American Indian. In *The Physical Anthropology of the American Indian*. The Viking Fund, Inc., New York.
1963. Analysis of the American Indian Dentition. In *Dental Anthropology*. Don Brothwell (Ed.), Pergamon Press, London. pp. 149–177.
1963. Dental Evolution and Culture. *Human Biology*. Vol. 35, No. 3, pp, 237–249.
1964. Aging Patterns in Teeth. *International Dental Journal*. Vol. 14, No. 3, pp. 376–390.

Dalton, Harry P., Marvin J. Allison, Alejandro Pezzia
1976. The Documentation of Communicable Diseases in Peruvian Mummies. *Medical College of Virginia Quarterly*, Vol. 12, No. 2, pp. 43–48.

Dechaume, M., L. Derobert, and J. Payen
1960. De la valeur de la determination de l'age par l'examen des dents en coupes minces. *Annales de Medecine Legale*, Vol. 40, pp. 165–167.

Denninger, Henri Stearns
1931. Osteitis Fibrosa in a Skeleton of a Prehistoric American Indian. *Archives of Pathology*, Vol. 11, pp. 939–947.
1933. Paleopathological Evidence of Paget's Disease. *Annals of Medical History*, New Series. Vol. 5, No. 1, pp. 73–81.

1935. Prehistoric Syphilitic Lesions. *Southwestern Medicine,* Vol. 19, pp. 202–204.

Densmore, Frances
1926–27. Use of Plants by the Chippewa Indians. *44th Annual Report of the Bureau of American Ethnology.* pp. 332–335.

Dockstader, F. J.
1954. The Kachina and the White Man. *Cranbrook Institute of Science, Bulletin 35,* p. 50, 123, 129. Bloomfield Hills, Michigan.

Enlow, Donald H.
1963. *Principles of Bone Remodeling.* Charles C Thomas, Springfield, Illinois.

Enlow, Donald H. and Sidney O. Brown
1956. A Comparative Histological Study of Fossil and Recent Bone Tissues. Part I. *Texas Journal of Science,* Vol. 8, No. 4, pp. 405–443.
1957. A comparative Histological Study of Fossil and Recent Bone Tissues, Part II. *Texas Journal of Science,* Vol. 9, No. 2, pp. 186–214.
1958. A Comparative Histological Study of Fossil and Recent Bone Tissues, Part III. *Texas Journal of Science,* Vol. 10, No. 3, pp. 187–230.

Epstein, Bernard S.
1962. *The Spine.* Lea and Febiger, Philadelphia.

Ericksen, Mary Frances
1973. *Age-Related Bone Remodeling in Three Aboriginal American Populations.* Ph.D. Dissertation. George Washington University.

Falk, A.
1958. A Follow-up of Skeletal Tuberculosis. *J. Bone Joint Surgery* (Amer), Vol. 40. p. 1162.

Fewkes, J. W.
1899–1900. Hopi Katchinas, *21st Annual Report of Bureau of American Ethnology,* p. 86.

Fisher, Alton K.
1935. Additional Paleopathological Evidence of Paget's Disease. *Annals of Medical History,* New Series, Vol. 7, No. 2, pp. 197–198.

Fisher, Alton K., Herbert W. Kuhn and George C. Adami
1931. Dental Pathology of the Prehistoric Indians of Wisconsin. *Bulletin of the Public Museum of the City of Milwaukee,* Vol. 10, No. 3, pp. 332–374.

Frost, H. M.
1959. Staining of Fresh, Undecalicified Thin Bone Sections. *Stain Technology,* Vol. 34, pp. 135–146.
1963. Mean Formation Time of Human Osteons. *Canadian Journal of Biochemistry and Physiology,* Vol. 41, No. 5, pp. 1307–1310.
1964. A Unique Histological Feature of Vitamin D Resistant Rickets Observed in Four Cases. *Acta Scandanavica Orthopedica,* Vol. 33, pp. 220–226.
1966. Morphometry of Bone in Palaeopathology. In *Human Palaeopathology,* Saul Jarcho (Ed.), Yale University Press, pp. 131–150.

Garcia-Frias, J. E.
1940. La Tuberculosis en los Antiquos Peruanos. *Actualidad Med Purana,* Vol. 5, p. 274.

Garn, Stanley M., Christabel G. Rohman, Betty Wagner and Werner Ascoli
1967. Continuing Bone Growth Throughout Life. *American Journal of Physical Anthropology,* Vol. 26, No. 3, pp. 313–317.

Garn, Stanley M. and Patricia M. Schwager
1967. Age Dynamics of Persistent Transverse Lines in the Tibia. *American Journal of Physical Anthropology,* Vol. 27, No. 3, pp. 357–377.

Gerszten, Enrique, Marvin Allison, Alejandro Pezzia, and David Klurfeld
1976. Thyroid Disease in a Peruvian Mummy. *Medical College of Virginia Quarterly,* Vol. 12, No. 2, pp. 52–53.

Gerszten, Enrique, Juan Munizaga, Marvin J. Allison and David Klurfeld
1976. Diaphragmatic Hernia of the Stomach in a Peruvian Mummy. *Bulletin of the New York Academy of Medicine,* 2nd Series, Vol. 52, No. 5, pp. 601–604.

Girdlestone, G. R.
1940. *Tuberculosis of Bone and Joint.* Oxford University Press, Inc., New York.

Glanville, Edward V.
1967. Perforation of the Coronoid-Olecranon Septum. *American Journal of Physical Anthropology,* Vol. 26, pp. 85–92.

Goff, C. W.
1967. Syphilis. In *Diseases in Antiquity.* Don Brothwell and A. T. Sandison (Eds.), Charles C Thomas, Springfield, pp. 279–294.

Graham, Daniel
1973. *The Use of X-ray Techniques in Forensic Investigations.* Churchill Livingstone, London. pp. 137–140.

Griffin, James B.
1960. A Hypothesis for the Prehistory of the Winnebago. In *Culture in History: Essays in Honor of Paul Radin.* Stanley Diamond (Ed.), Columbia University Press, N.Y., pp. 809–865.

Griffin, James B. (Ed.)
1952. *Archeology of Eastern United States.* University of Chicago Press, Chicago.

Guri, J. P.
1947. Formation and Significance of Vertebral Ankylosis in Tuberculous Spines. *J. Bone Joint Surgery* (Amer), Vol. 29.

Gustafson, Gosta
1950. Age Determinations on Teeth. *The Journal of the American Dental Association,* Vol. 41, pp. 45–54.

Hackett, C. J.
1951. *Bone Lesions of Yaws in Uganda.* Blackwell Scientific Publications, Oxford.

Hall, Robert L.
1962. *The Archaeology of Carcajou Point, with an Intepretation of the Development of Oneota Culture in Wisconsin,* 2 Vols. University of Wisconsin Press, Madison.

Hallock, H. and J. B. Jones
1954. Tuberculosis of the Spine. *J Bone Joint Surgery* (Amer), Vol. 36, p. 219.

Hamilton, Henry W.
1952. The Spiro Mound. *The Missouri Archaeologist,* Columbia. Vol. 14.

Harn, Alan D.
1966. *Skeletons and Artifacts from the Dickson Cemetery Mounds,* Illinois State Museum Society, Springfield, Illinois.

Harris, James E. and Kent R. Weeks
1973. *X-Raying the Pharaohs.* Charles Scribner's Sons, New York.

Harris, R. I.
1949. Osteological Evidence of Disease Amongst the Huron Indians. *University of Toronto Medical Journal,* Vol. XXXVII, No. 2, pp. 71–75.

Harris, R. I. and H. S. Coulthard
1942. Prognosis in Bone and Joint Tuberculosis. *J Bone Joint Surgery* (Amer), Vol. 24, p. 385.

Harvey, Warren and Henry W. Noble
1968. Defects on the Lingual Surface of the Mandible Near the Angle. *British Journal of Oral Surgery,* Vol. 6, No. 2, pp. 75–83.

Hinkle, C. L.
1957. Developmental Affections of the Skeleton Characterized by Osteosclerosis. *Clinical Orthopaedics,* No. 9, J. B. Lippincott Co., Philadelphia.

Hinsdale, W. B. and Emerson F. Greenman
1936. Perforated Indian Crania in Michigan, *Occasional Contributions, Museum of Anthropology,* No. 5. University of Michigan, Ann Arbor.

History of Fulton County, Illinois. Author unknown.
1879. Chap. XI. Charles C. Chapman & Co., Peoria.

Hohenthal, William D. and Sheilagh Thompson Brooks
1960. An Archaeological Scaphocephal from California. *American Journal of Physical Anthropology,* Vol. 18, No. 1, pp. 59–68.

Holder, Preston and T. D. Stewart
1958. Anthropology, A Complete Find of Filed Teeth from the Cahokia Mounds in Illinois. *Journal of the Washington Academy of Science,* Vol. 48, No. 11, pp. 349–357.

Hollander, J. L. (Ed.)
1966. *Arthritis.* Classification, pp. 24–26; Radiology, pp. 136–141; Rheumatoid by Leon Sokoloff, Chapter 13; Ankylosing Spondylitis by L. W. Boland, Chapter 39. Lea & Febiger, Philadelphia.

Holmes, W. H.
1882–1883. Ancient Pottery of the Mississippi Valley. *4th Annual Report of the Bureau of American Ethnology,* pp. 425–426.
1898–1899. Aboriginal Pottery of Eastern United States. *20th Annual Report of the Bureau of American Ethnology,* p. 95.

Hooton, E. A.
1930. *Indians of Pecos Pueblo.* Yale University Press, New Haven.

Hoyme, Lucile
1962. Human Skeletal Remains from the Tollifero and Clarkville Sites. *Bureau of American Ethnology, Bulletin 182,* pp. 329–400.

Hrdlicka, Ales
1908. Physiological and Medical Observations. *Bureau of American Ethnology, Bulletin 34,* pp. 79, 208–212, 238–252.
1909. Tuberculosis among Certain Indian Tribes. *Bureau of American Ethnology, Bulletin 42.*
1913. A Report on a Collection of Crania and Bones from Sorrel Bayou, Iberville Parish, Louisiana. *Journal of the Academy of Natural Sciences,* Vol. 16, p. 97.
1914. Pathology of the Ancient Peruvians, *Smithsonian Miscellaneous Collections,* Vol. XLI, No. 18.
1939. Trepanation Among Prehistoric People. *Ciba Symposia,* Vol. 1, No. 5, pp. 170–178.

Hunter, King B.
1968. Preliminary Report. Klunk Site Skeletons. in "Hopewell and Woodland Site Archaeology in Illinois," *Illinois Archaeological Survey, Bulletin 6,* pp. 125–128.
1968. "The Genetic, Temporal and Spacial Relationships of the Hopewellian Populations of the Illinois Valley." Unpublished Ph.D. Dissertation. Indiana University, Bloomington, Indiana.

Irani, R. N. and Mary S. Sherman
1963. The Pathological Anatomy of Club Foot. *J Bone Joint Surgery* (Amer), Vol. 45, No. 1, pp. 45–52.

Jackson, F. E., MC. U.S. Navy
1966. The Pathophysiology of Head Injuries. *Ciba Symposia,* Vol. 18, No. 3, pp. 67–73.

Jaffe, Henry L.
1958. *Tumors and Tumorous Conditions of the Bones and Joints.* Lea and Febiger, Philadelphia. p. 76.

Johnson, Lent C.
1959. Kinetics of Osteoarthritis. *Laboratory Investigation,* Vol. 8, pp. 1223–1238.
1964. Joint Remodeling as the Basis for Osteoarthritis. *Journal of the American Veterinary Association,* Vol. 141, No. 10, pp. 1237–1241.

Jones, Joseph
1876. Explorations of the Aboriginal Remains of Tennessee. *Smithsonian Contributions to Knowledge,* Vol. 22 (259), Washington.

Jowsey, J.
1960. Age Changes in Human Bone. *Clinical Orthopaedics,* Vol. 17, pp. 210–217.

Jowsey, J., P. J. Kelly, B. L. Riggs, A. J. Bianco, D. A. Scholz and J. Gershon-Cohen
1965. *Quantitative Microradiographic Studies of Normal and Osteoporotic Bone.* Journal of Bone and Joint Surgery, Vol. 47A, pp. 785–806.

Judd, N. M.
1954. The Material Culture of Pueblo Bonito. *Smithsonian Miscellaneous Collections,* Vol. 124.

Karsner, H. T.
1955. *Human Pathology.* J. B. Lippincott Co., Philadelphia, pp. 448–454, 798–799.

Kelso, Jack and George Ewing
1962. *Introduction to Physical Anthropology Laboratory Manual.* Pruett Press, Inc., Boulder, Colorado.

Kerley, Ellis R.
1965. The Microscopic Determination of Age in Human Bone. *American Journal of Physical Anthropology,* Vol. 23, pp. 149–164.

Kidder, A. V. and S. J. Guernsey
1919. Archaeological Explorations in Northeastern Arizona. *Bureau of American Ethnology,* Bulletin 65, p. 195.

Knaggs, R. L.
1926. *Diseases of Bone.* William Wood & Co., New York.

Krogman, Wilton Marion
1962. *The Human Skeleton in Forensic Medicine.* Charles C Thomas, Springfield, Illinois.

Lafond, E. M.
1958. An Analysis of Adult Skeletal Tuberculosis. *J Bone Joint Surgery* (Amer), Vol. 40, p. 348.

Langford, G.
1927. The Fisher Mound Group. *American Anthropologist,* Vol. 29, No. 3.

Lester, Charles W. and Harry L. Shapiro
1968. Vertebral Arch Defects in the Lumbar Vertebrae of Pre-historic American Eskimos. *American Journal of Physical Anthropology,* Vol. 28, No. 1, pp. 43–47.

Lichtor, J. and A. A. Lichtor
1957. Paleopathological Evidence Suggesting Pre-Columbian Tuberculosis of the Spine. *J Bone Joint Surgery* (Amer), Vol. 39-A, p. 1398.

Linne, S.
1943. Humpbacks in Ancient America. *Ethnos,* Vol. 8, p. 161.

Lister, S.
1932. Tuberculosis in South African Natives. The *South African Institute for Medical Research,* Johannesburg, Vol. 5, No. 30.

Luck, J. Vernon
1950. *Bone and Joint Diseases.* Charles C Thomas, Springfield, Illinois.

Luntz, Lester L. and Phyllys Luntz
1973. *Handbook for Dental Identification.* J. P. Lippincott Co., Philadelphia. pp. 88–90.

MacCurdy, G. G.
1923. Human Skeletal Remains from the Highlands of Peru. *American Journal of Physical Anthropology,* Vol. 6, No. 3, p. 264.

Maresh, Marion M.
1955. Linear Growth of Long Bones of Extremities from Infancy Through Adolescence. *Diseases of Children,* Vol. 89, pp. 725–746.

McDonald, S. E.
1950. The Crable Site, Fulton County, Illinois. *Journal of the Illinois State Archaeological Society,* Vol. 7, No. 4, pp. 16–18.

McGregor, J. C. and William H. Wadlow
1951. A Trephined Skull from Illinois. *American Anthropologist,* Vol. 53, No. 1, pp. 148–152.

Merbs, Charles F. and William H. Wilson
1960. *Anomalies and Pathologies of the Sadlermiut Eskimo Vertebral Column.* Part I, Bulletin No. 180. National Museum of Canada, Ottawa.

Meschan, Isadore
1959. *Normal Radiographic Anatomy.* W. B. Saunders Co., Philadelphia. pp. 1–24.

Michaelis, Lorenz
1930. Vergleichende Mikroskopische Untersuchungen an Rezenten, Historischen und Fossilen Menschichen Knochen. Zugleich ein Beitrag zur Geschichte der Syphilis, Fischer, Jena.

Mielke, James H., George J. Armelagos and Dennis P. Van Geryen
1972. Trabecular Involution in Femoral Heads of a Pre-historic (X-Group) Population from Sudanese Nubia. *American Journal of Physical Anthropology,* Vol. 36, No. 1, pp. 39–44.

Moldawer, Marc and Erwin R. Rabin
1966. Polyostotic Fibrous Dysplasia with Thyrotoxicosis. *Archives of Internal Medicine,* Vol. 118, pp. 379–384.

Moodie, Roy L.
1918. Studies in Paleopathology, Pathological Evidences of Disease Among Ancient Races of Man and Extinct Animals. *Surgery, Gynecology and Obstetrics,* pp. 498–510.
1923a. *The Antiquity of Disease.* The University of Chicago Press, Chicago.
1923b. *Paleopathology:* An Introduction to the Study of Ancient Evidences of Disease. University of Illinois Press, Urbana.
1926. Studies in Paleopathology, XIII: the Elements of the Haversian System in Normal and Pathological Structures among Fossil Vertebrates. *Biologia Generalis,* Vol. II, No. 1/2, pp. 63–95.

Mooney, James
1900. Scalping. *19th Annual Report of Bureau of American Ethnology.* Pt. I, pp. 47, 50–53, 208–209.
1910. Scalping. Handbook of American Indians. *Bureau of American Ethnology, Bulletin 30,* Part 2, p. 482.

Mooney, James and Frans M. Olbrechts
1932. The Swimmer Manuscript. *Bureau of American Ethnology, Bulletin 99,* pp. 71–72.

Moore, C.
1913. Some Aboriginal Sites in Louisiana and in Arkansas. *Journal of the Academy of Natural Sciences,* Philadelphia, Vol. 16, p. 13.

Moorehead, Warren K.
1932. *Etowah Papers.* Yale University Press, New Haven.

Morse, Dan
1944. The Chest X-ray. *Diseases of the Chest,* Vol. X, No. 6, p. 5.
1961. Prehistoric Tuberculosis in America. *American Review of Respiratory Diseases,* Vol. 83, No. 4, pp. 489–504.
1967. Tuberculosis. Chapter 19. In *Diseases in Antiquity.* Brothwell and Sandison (Ed.), Charles C Thomas, Springfield, Illinois.
1967. Two Cases of Possible Treponema Infection in Prehistoric America. Technical Series No. 7. *Miscellaneous Papers in Paleopathology:* I, William D. Wade (Ed), Museum of Northern Arizona, Flagstaff, pp. 48–60.
1969. The Origin of Treponematosis. *Proceedings of the Peoria Academy of Science,* Vol. 2, pp. 27–32.
1973. *Pathology and Abnormalities.* In Nodena, Arkansas Archaeological Survey, Research Series, No. 4, (Ed.) Dan F. Morse, pp. 48–50.

Morse, Dan, Donald Crusoe and H. G. Smith
1976. Forensic Archaeology. *Journal of Forensic Sciences,* Vol. 21, pp. 323–332.

Morse, Dan, Don R. Brothwell and Peter J. Ucko
1964. Tuberculosis in Ancient Egypt. *American Review of Respiratory Diseases,* Vol. 90, No. 4, pp. 524–541.

Morse, Dan, George Schoenbeck and Dan F. Morse
1953. Fiedler Site. *Journal of the Illinois State Archaeological Society,* Vol. 3, pp. 34–46.

Morse, Dan F.
1958. Some Preliminary Notes on a Red Ocher Mound at the Morse Site. *Central States Archaeological Journal*, Vol. 5, No. 1, pp. 16–17.
1960. The Southern Cult. The Crable Site, Fulton County, Illinois. *Central States Archaeological Journal*, Vol. 7, No. 4, pp. 124–135.
1963. Steuben Village and Mounds. *Anthropological Papers*, No. 21, Museum of Anthropology, University of Michigan, Ann Arbor.
1967. The Robinson Site and Shell Mound Archaic Culture in the Middle South. Unpublished Ph.D. Thesis, University of Michigan, Ann Arbor.

Morse, Dan F. and Don F. Dickson
1956. Prehistoric Pathology. *Central States Archaeological Journal*, Vol. 2, No. 4, pp. 143–151.

Morse, Dan F. and Phyllis Morse
1964. 1962 Excavations at the Morse Site: A Red Ocher Cemetery in the Illinois Valley. *The Wisconsin Archeologist*, New Series, Vol. 45, No. 2, pp. 79–87.

Morse, Dan F., Phyllis Morse and Merrill Emmons
1961. The Southern Cult. The Emmons Site, Fulton County, Illinois. *Central States Archaeological Journal*, Vol. 8, No. 4, pp. 124–140.

Mosely, John E.
1963. Bone Changes in Hematologic Disorders, Grune & Stratton, New York.
1966. Radiographic Studies in Hematologic Bone Disease. In *Human Paleopathology*, Saul Jarcho (Ed.). Yale University Press, New Haven. pp. 120–130.

Moss, Martin and Allan C. Levey
1966. The Traumatic Bone Cyst: Report of Three Cases. *Journal of the American Dental Association*, Vol. 72, pp. 397–402.

Munizaga, Juan, Marvin J. Allison, Enrique Gerszten and David M. Klurfeld
1975. Pneumoconiosis in Chilean Miners of the 16th Century. *Bulletin of the New York Academy of Medicine*, 2nd Series, Vol. 51, No. 11, pp. 1281–1293.

Myerding, H. W.
1944. Chronic Scherosing Osteitis. *South. Clin. North America*, Vol. 24, p. 762.

Nalbandian, J.
1959. Age Changes in Human Teeth. *Journal of Dental Research*, Vol. 38, pp. 681–682.

Nalbandian, J. and R. F. Sognnaes
1960. Structural Age Changes in Human Teeth. In Aging. Nathan W. Shock (Ed.) , *American Association for the Advancement of Science*, Vol. 65, Washington, D.C., pp. 367–382.

National Council on Radiation Protection and Measurements.
1968. *Medical X-ray and Gamma-Ray Protection for Energies up to 10 MeV.* Report 33, NCRP, Washington, D. C.

Nestmann, Friedrich
1928. Histologische Untersuchungen an Syphilitisch Veranderten Tibien. *Archiv fur orthopadische und Unfall-Chirurgie*, Vol. 26, pp. 237–252.

Neumann, Georg K.
1940. Evidence for the Antiquity of Scalping from Central Illinois. *American Antiquity*, Vol. V, No. 4, pp. 287–289.
1942. Types of Artificial Deformation in the Eastern United States. *American Antiquity*, Vol. VII, No. 3, pp. 306–310.
1952. Archeology and Race in the American Indian. In *Archeology of Eastern United States*, James B. Griffin (Ed.), University of Chicago Press, Chicago, pp. 13–14.
1960. Origins of the Indians of the Middle Mississippi Area. *Proceedings of the Indiana Academy of Science for 1959*, Vol. 69, pp. 66–68. Bloomington, Indiana.
1961. *Laboratory Manual of Bioanthropology.* Department of Anthropology, University of Indiana, Bloomington, Indiana.

Neumann, Georg K. and Melvin L. Fowler
1952. Hopewellian Sites in the Lower Wabash Valley. In "Hopewellian Communities in Illinois," Thorne Deuel (Ed.), *Illinois State Museum Scientific Papers*, Vol. V, p. 209.

Neumann, Holm W.
1967. The Paleopathology of the Archaic Modoc Rock Shelter Inhabitants. *Illinois State Museum Reports of Investigations*, No. 11, Springfield, Illinois.

Oakley, K. P., Winifred Brook, A. Roger Akester and Don Brothwell
1959. Contributions on Trepanning or Trephination in Ancient and Modern Times. *Man*, Vol. LIX, pp. 92–96.

O'Bannon, L. G.
1957. Evidence of Tuberculosis of the Spine from a Mississippi Box Burial. *Tennessee Archaeologist*, Vol. 13, No. 2.

Olson, Ronald L.
1930. Chumash Prehistory. *University of California Publications in American Archaeology and Ethnology*, Vol. 28, No. 1, pp. 1–21.

Ortner, Donald J.
1968. Description and Classification of Degenerative Bone Changes in the Distal Joint Surfaces of the Humerus. *American Journal of Physical Anthropology*, Vol. 28, No. 2, pp. 139–155.
1975. Aging Effects on Osteon Remodeling. *Calcified Tissue Research*, Vol. 18, pp. 27–36.
In Press. Microscopic and Molecular Biology of Human Compact Bone: Anthropological Perspective. Submitted to *American Journal of Physical Anthropology*.

Otis, George A. and D. L. Huntington
The Medical and Surgical History of the War of the Rebellion.
1875. *Surgical History.* Part 1. Vol. 2.
1877. *Surgical History.* Part 2. Vol 1.
1883. *Surgical History.* Part 3. Vol. 2.
Prepared under the direction of the Surgeon General, Washington, D.C.

Owen, Richard
1840–1845. *Odontography.* Hippolyte. Bailliere, London.

Pales, D. L.
1930. *Paleopathologie Tuberculose Pre-Historique.* Masson & Cie, Editeurs, Paris. Ch. 10, pp. 226–247.

Pancoast, Henry K., Eugene P. Pendergrass and J. Parsons Schaeffer
1940. *Head and Neck in Roentgen Diagnosis.* Charles C Thomas, Springfield, Illinois.

Pansky, Ben and Earl Lawrence House
1969. *Review of Gross Anatomy,* 2nd edition. The MacMillan Company, New York.

Parsons, E. C.
1938. The Humpbacked Flute Player of the Southwest. *American Anthropology,* Vol. 40, p. 337.

Perino, Gregory
1966. The Bank's Village Site. *Missouri Archaeological Society Memoir,* No. 4, Columbia.
1968. The Pete Klunk Mound Group. In "Hopewell and Woodland Site Archaeology in Illinois," James A. Brown (Ed.). *Illinois Archaeological Survey,* Bulletin 6, pp. 9–24.

Perkins, Raymond W.
1965. The Frederick Site. In "Middle Woodland Sites in Illinois," Elaine Bluhm Herold (Ed.), *Illinois Archaeological Survey,* Bulletin 5, pp. 69–96.

Perou, Maurice L.
1964. *Cranial Hyperostosis.* Charles C Thomas, Springfield, Illinois. pp. 35–39.

Post, P. W. and F. Daniels
1969. Histological and Histochemical Examination of American Indian Scalps, Mummies, and a Shrunken Head. *American Journal of Physical Anthropology,* Vol. 30, No. 2, pp. 269–293.

Primer on the Rheumatic Disease.
1959. Prepared by a Committee of the American Rheumatism Association. Arthritis and Rheumatism Foundation, New York.

Pugh, David G.
1958. *Roentgenologic Diagnosis of Diseases of Bone.* Williams and Wilkins, Baltimore.

Putschar, Walter G. J.
1966. Problems in the Pathology and Palaeopathology of Bone. In *Human Palaeopathology.* Saul Jarcho (Ed.), Yale University Press, pp. 57–65.

Quekett, John
1849. On the Intimate Structure of Bone . . . and XI Additional Observations . . . *Transactions of the Royal Microscopic Society of London,* Vol. II, pp. 46–64.
1852. *A Practical Treatise on the Use of the Microscope,* 2nd edition, H. Bailliere, London.

Requena, A.
1945. Evidencia de Tuberculosis en la America Pre-Columbian. *Acta Venezolana, Caracas,* Tomo 1, No. 2.

Riesenfeld, Alphonse
1956. Multiple Infraorbital Ethmoidal and Mental Foramina in the Races of Man. *American Journal of Physical Anthropology,* Vol. 14, No. 1, pp. 85–100.

Ritchie, W. A.
1944. *The Pre-Iroquoian Occupations of New York State.* Rochester Museum of Arts and Sciences, Rochester, New York.
1952. Pathological Evidence Suggesting Pre-Columbian Tuberculosis in New York State. *American Journal of Physical Anthropology,* Vol. 10, p. 305.

Ritvo, M.
1955. *Bone and Joint X-ray Diagnosis.* Lea and Febiger, Philadelphia.

Roberts, F. H. H.
1932. The Village of the Great Kivas. *Bureau of American Ethnology,* Bulletin III, p. 150.

Rossencrantz, E., A. Piscitelli and F. C. Bost
1941. An Analytical Study of Bone and Joint Lesions in Relation to Chronic Pulmonary Tuberculosis. *J Bone Joint Surgery* (Amer), Vol. 23, p. 630.

Ross, John A. and R. W. Galloway
1963. *A Handbook of Radiography.* H. K. Lewis and Co., Ltd., London, pp. 1–30.

Rowe, G. G. and M. B. Roche
1953. Etiology of Separate Neural Arch. *J Bone Joint Surgery* (Amer), Vol. 35A, pp. 102–110.

Rubin, Phillip
1964. *Modeling Sketches and Skeletons in the Dynamic Classification of Bone Dysplasias.* Year Book Medical Publishers, Chicago.

Ruffer, Marc Armand
1910. Note on the Presence of "Bilharzia Haematobia" in Egyptian Mummies of the Twentieth Dynasty (1250–1000 B.C.). *The British Medical Journal,* Vol. 1, p. 16.
1912. On Osseous Lesions in Ancient Egyptians. *Journal of Pathology and Bacteriology,* Vol. XVI, pp. 439–465.
1914. On a tumour of the pelvis dating from the Roman times (250 A.D.) and found in Egypt. *Journal of Pathology and Bacteriology,* Vol. XVIII, pp. 480–484.
1921. *Studies in the Palaeopathology of Egypt.* Roy L. Moodie (Ed.). University of Chicago Press.

Salomon, Carl D. and Nicu Haas
1967. Histological and Histochemical Observations on Undecalcified Sections of Ancient Bones From Excavations in Israel. *Israel Journal of Medical Science,* Vol. 3, pp. 747–754.

Sandison, A. T.
1968. Pathological Changes in the Skeletons of Earlier Populations Due to Acquired Disease, and Difficulties in their Interpretations. In *The Skeletal Biology of Earlier Human Populations.* D. R. Brothwell (Ed.). Pergamon Press, London, pp. 205–243.
1970. The Study of Mummified and Dried Human Tissues. In *Science in Archaeology.* Don Brothwell and Eric Higgs (Eds.). Praeger, New York, pp. 490–502.

Sarat, B. G. and D. M. Laskin
1962. *Diagnosis and Surgical Management of Diseases of the Temporomandibular Joint.* Charles C Thomas, Springfield, Illinois. p. 27.

Sedlin, Elias D., Antonio R. Villanueva and Harold M. Frost
1963. Age Variations in the Specific Surface of Howship's Lacunae as an Index of Human Bone

Resorption. *Anatomical Record,* Vol. 146, No. 3, pp. 201–207.

Shands, Alfred Rives
1952. *Handbook of Orthopaedic Surgery,* C. V. Mosby, St. Louis.

Shaw, A. F. B.
1938. Histological Study of Mummy of Har-mose, Singer of Eighteenth Dynasty (circa 1490 B.C.). *Journal of Pathology and Bacteriology,* Vol. 47, pp. 115–123.

Siegrist, H. E.
1951. *A History of Medicine.* Oxford University Press, New York.

Simpson, A. M.
1939. *The Kingston Village Site.* The Peoria Academy of Science, Peoria, Illinois.

Singh, I. J. and D. L. Gunberg
1970. Estimation of Age at Death in Human Males from Quantitative Histology of Bone Fragments. *American Journal of Physical Anthropology,* Vol. 33, No. 3, pp. 373–381.

Smith, Hale G.
1951. The Crable Site. Fulton County, Illinois. *Anthropological Papers, Museum of Anthropology,* University of Michigan, Ann Arbor. No. 7.

Smyth, Charley J.
1963. Chairman Editorial Committee—Rheumatism and Arthritis Foundation. Fifteenth Rheumatism Review. *Annals of Internal Medicine,* Vol. 59, No. 5, Part II, Suppl. 4.

Snow, Charles E.
1941. Anthropological Studies at Moundville. *Alabama Museum of Natural History, Museum Paper 15.* Geological Survey of Alabama, University, Alabama.
1943. Two Prehistoric Indian Dwarf Skeletons from Moundville. *Alabama Museum of Natural History, Museum Paper 21.* Geological Survey of Alabama, University, Alabama.
1948. Indian Knoll Skeletons. *Reports in Anthropology,* Vol. IV, No. 3, Part II. University of Kentucky, Lexington.

Sognnaes, Reidar F.
1956. Histologic Evidence of Developmental Lesions in Teeth Originating from Paleolithic, Prehistoric, and Ancient Man. *American Journal of Pathology,* Vol. XXXII, No. 2, pp. 547–577.
1963. Dental Hard Tissue Destruction with Special Reference to Idiopathic Erosions. In *Mechanisms of Hard Tissue Destruction,* R. Sognnaes (Ed.), Publication No. 75 of the AAAS, Washington, pp. 91–153.

Staheli, Lynn T., Charles C. Church and Byron H. Ward
1968. Infantile Cortical Hyperostosis. *Journal of the American Medical Association,* Vol. 203, No. 6, pp. 384–386.

Steinbock, R. Ted
1976. Paleopathological Diagnosis and Interpretation. Charles C Thomas, Springfield.

Steindler, A.
1952. Postgraduate Lectures on Orthopedic Diagnosis and Indications. *Tuberculosis of the Skeletal System,* Section A, Vol. III. Charles C Thomas, Springfield, Illinois.

Stern, E. W. and A. E. Stearn
1945. *The Effect of Smallpox on the Destiny of the Amerindian.* Bruce Humphries, Inc., Boston.

Stern, Frances
1936. *Applied Dietetics.* Williams & Wilkins Co., Baltimore. pp. 156–157.

Stewart, T. D.
1940. Skeletal Remains from the Whitewater District, Eastern Arizona. *Bureau of American Ethnology, Bulletin 126,* pp. 153–176.
1941. Skeletal Remains from the Peachtree Site, North Carolina. *Bureau of American Ethnology,* Bulletin 131, pp. 81–99.
1950. Pathological Changes in South American Indian Skeletal Remains. Handbook of South American Indians. *Bureau of American Ethnology,* Bulletin 143, Vol. 6, pp. 49–52.
1953. Skeletal Remains from Zaculeu Guatemala: In *The Ruins of Zaculeu Guatemala,* by Richard B. Woodbury and Aubrey S. Trik. Vol. I, pp. 295–311. Vol. II, p. 455, United Fruit Co., Hartford, Conn.
1956. Examination of the Possibility that Certain Characters Predispose to Defects in the Lumbar Arch. *Clinical Orthopaedics.* J. B. Lippincott Co., Philadelphia. No. 8, pp. 44–46.
1958. Stone Age Skull Surgery. *Annual Report of the Board of Regents of the Smithsonian Institution for 1957,* pp. 469–491.
1958. The Rate of Development of Vertebral Osteoarthritis in American Whites and its Significance in Skeletal Age Identification. *The Leech,* Vol. XXVIII, No. 3, 4 and 5, pp. 144–151.
1960. Description of Skeletal Remains from Doniphan and Scott Counties, Kansas. *Bureau of American Ethnology, Bulletin 174,* p. 672.
1966. Some Problems in Human Paleopathology. In *Human Paleopathology,* Yale University Press, New Haven.

Stewart, T. D. and Alexander Spoehr
1952. Evidence of the Paleopathology of Yaws. *Bulletin of the History of Medicine,* Vol. XXVI, No. 6.

Stevenson, Matilda Coxe
1901–1902. The Zuni Indians. *23rd Annual Report of the Bureau of American Ethnology,* pp. 391–392.

Stone, Eric
1962. Medicine Among the American Indians. *Clio Medica.* Hafner Publishing Co., New York.

Stothers, David M. and James F. Metress
1975. A System for the Description and Analysis of Pathological Changes in Prehistoric Skeletons. *Ossa,* Vol. 2, pp. 3–9.

Stout, Samuel D. and Steven L. Teitelbaum
1976. Histological Analysis of Undecalcified Thin Sections of Archaeological Bone. *American Journal of Physical Anthropology,* Vol. 44, No. 2, pp. 263–269.

Swedlund, Alan C. and William D. Wade
1972. *Laboratory Methods in Physical Anthropology.* Prescott College Press, Prescott, Arizona.

Tennessee Division of State Parks
No date. *Chucalissa Indian Museum*, Pamphlet. Memphis, Tennessee.

Titterington, Paul E.
1938. *The Cahokia Mound Group and its Village Site Material*. Published by the Author, St. Louis.

Tobin, William J. and Dale Stewart
1953. Gross Osteopathology of Arthritis. *Clinical Orthopaedics*, J. B. Lippincott Co., Philadelphia. No. 2, pp. 167–183.

Turek, Samual L.
1959. *Orthopaedics*. J. B. Lippincott Co., Philadelphia.

Ubelaker, Douglas H.
1974. Reconstruction of Demographic Profiles from Ossuary Skeletal Samples. *Smithsonian Contributions to Anthropology*, No. 18, Washington.

Valentine, R. G.
1912. *Eighty-first Annual Report of the Commissioner of Indian Affairs*, U. S. Department of Interior. p. 169.

Van Gerven, Dennis P.
1973. Thickness and Area Measurements as Parameters of Skeletal Involution of the Humerus, Femur, and Tibia. *Journal of Gerontology*, Vol. 28, No. 1, pp. 40–45.

Van Gerven, Dennis P. and George J. Armelagos
1970. Cortical Involution in Prehistoric Mississippian Femora. *Journal of Gerontology*, Vol. 25, No. 1, pp. 20–22.

Villanueva, Antonio R., Elias D. Sedlin, and Harold M. Frost
1963. Variations in Osteoblastic Activity with Age by the Osteoid Seam Index. *Anatomical Record*, Vol. 146, No. 3, pp. 209–213.

Walker, G. F.
1976. *The Computer and the Law: Coordinate Analysis of Skull Shape and Possible Methods of Postmortem Identification*. Journal of Forensic Sciences, Vol. 21, No. 3, pp. 357–366.

Webb, Clarence H.
1944. Dental Abnormalities as Found in the American Indian. *American Journal of Orthodontics and Oral Surgery*, Vol. 9, pp. 474–486.

Webb, G. B.
1936. Tuberculosis. *Clio Medica*. Paul B. Hoeber, New York.

Weber. M.
1927. Schliffe von Mazerierten Röhrenknochen und ihre Bedeutung für die Unterscheidung der Syphilis und Osteomyelitis von der Osteodystrophis fibrosa sowie für die Untersuchung Fraglich Syphilitischer Prähistorischer Knochen. *Beiträge zur pathologischen Anatomie und zur allgemeinen Pathologie*, Jena, Vol. 78, pp. 441–511.

Weinmann, J. P. and M. D. Sicher
1947. *Bone and Bones*. C. V. Mosby Co., St. Louis.

Weiss, Pedro
1958. Osteologia Cultural. Practicas Cefalicas. Cabaza Trofeos-Trepanaciones-Cauterizaciones. La

Parte. *Anales De La Facultad De Medicina*, Lima, Peru.

Wells, Calvin
1964. *Bones, Bodies and Disease*. Frederick A. Praeger, New York.
1967. A New Approach to Paleopathology: Harris's Lines. In *Diseases in Antiquity*, Brothwell and Sandison (Ed.), Charles C Thomas, Springfield, Illinois. Chapter 30, pp. 390–404.

Whitney, W. F.
1886. Notes on the Anomalies, Injuries and Diseases of the Bones of the Native Races of North America. *Annual Reports of the Peabody Museum of American Archaeology and Ethnology*, Vol. III, Nos. 5 and 6, p. 433.

Williams, Herbert U.
1926. Human Paleopathology. *Arch. Pathology*, Vol. 7, pp. 839–902.
1927. Gross and Microscopic Anatomy of Two Peruvian Mummies. *Archives of Pathology*, Vol. 4, No. 1, pp. 26–33.
1929a. Human Paleopathology: With Some Original Observations on Symmetrical Osteoporosis of the Skull. *Archives of Pathology*, Vol. 7, No. 4, pp. 839–902.
1929b. Symmetrical Osteoporosis of the Cranium. *The American Journal of Pathology*, Vol. 5, No. 5, pp. 524–525.
1932. The Origin and Antiquity of Syphilis: the Evidence from Diseased Bones. *Archives of Pathology*, Vol. 13, No. 5, pp. 779–814; No. 6, pp. 931–983.
1935. Pathology of Yaws. *Arch. Pathology*, Vol. 20, pp. 596–630.

Wilson, Gale E.
1927. A Study in American Paleohistology. *The American Naturalist*, Vol. 61, No. 667, pp. 555–565.

Wilson, Thomas
1901. Arrow Wounds, *American Anthropologist*, New Series, Vol. 3, pp. 513–531.

Wiltse, Leon L.
1957. Etiology of Spondylolisthesis. *Clinical Orthopaedics*, J. B. Lippincott Co., Philadelphia, No. 10, pp. 48–60.

Yeatman, G. W.
1971. Preservation of Chondrocyte Ultrastructure in an Aleutian Mummy. *Bulletin of the New York Academy of Medicine*, Vol. 47, pp. 104–108.

Zariquiey, Manuel O.
1958. Magicians and Meningiomas. *Medical Radiography and Photography*, Eastman Kodak Co., Rochester. Vol. 34, No. 3, p. 70.

Zimmerman, Michael R.
1972. Histological Examination of Experimentally Mummified Tissues. *American Journal of Physical Anthropology*, Vol. 37, No. 2, pp. 271–280.

Zimmerman, M. R., G. W. Yeatman, H. Sprinz, and W. P. Titterington
1971. Examination of an Aleutian Mummy. *Bulletin of the New York Academy of Medicine*, Vol. 47, pp. 80–103.

PLATE 1

DOCUMENTED HISTORIC DRIED BONE PATHOLOGY

A. Section through a lumbar vertebra of a patient who had Pagot's disease, showing enlarged vertebral body and diminution in size of neural canal. (Knaggs 1926, p. 303)

B. Osteogenesis Imperfecta. Showing bending deformities of long bones due to many fractures during lifetime. Male, age 68. Royal College of Surgeon's Museum Collection, No. 4172.1. (Knaggs 1926: 385)

C. Osteitis of frontal bone and perforation of nasal bone and palate in a known syphilitic prostitute. Age 30. Royal College of Surgeon's Museum Collection, General Pathology Section No. 1018.1. (Knaggs 1926:97)

D. Charcot's joint showing excessive callous and hyperplastic enlargement of knee and ankle joints. Most common cause is syphilis. Royal College of Surgeon's Museum Collection, No. 4578.1. (Knaggs 1926: 114)

E. Skull of case of Leontiasis Ossea. (Knaggs 1926:339. Knaggs also shows photograph of a Peruvian skull with Leontiasis Ossea.)

F. View of skull of a 17-year-old female whose skeleton was found by Indiana State Police near Indianapolis. Identification was made by Dr. Georg Neumann through the presence of only 11 thoracic vertebrae and a swelling of the left parietal bone. Hospital records revealed that, soon after birth, the girl had an infected hematoma over the left parietal area from which she recovered. Examination of specimens shows there is a raised area of new bone formation covering almost the entire left parietal bone and extending into the occipital and right parietal. The raised area is 3 mm. thicker at its highest point and the surface is roughened and covered with many tiny and well-healed holes. The borders of the affected area are sharply demarcated. This demonstrates bone reaction caused by adjacent soft tissue infection. *Photograph, courtesy Indiana State Police.*

G. Osteoarthritis involving pubic arch and sacroiliac and lumbosacral areas. (Knaggs 1926:176) See also Plate 11,D.

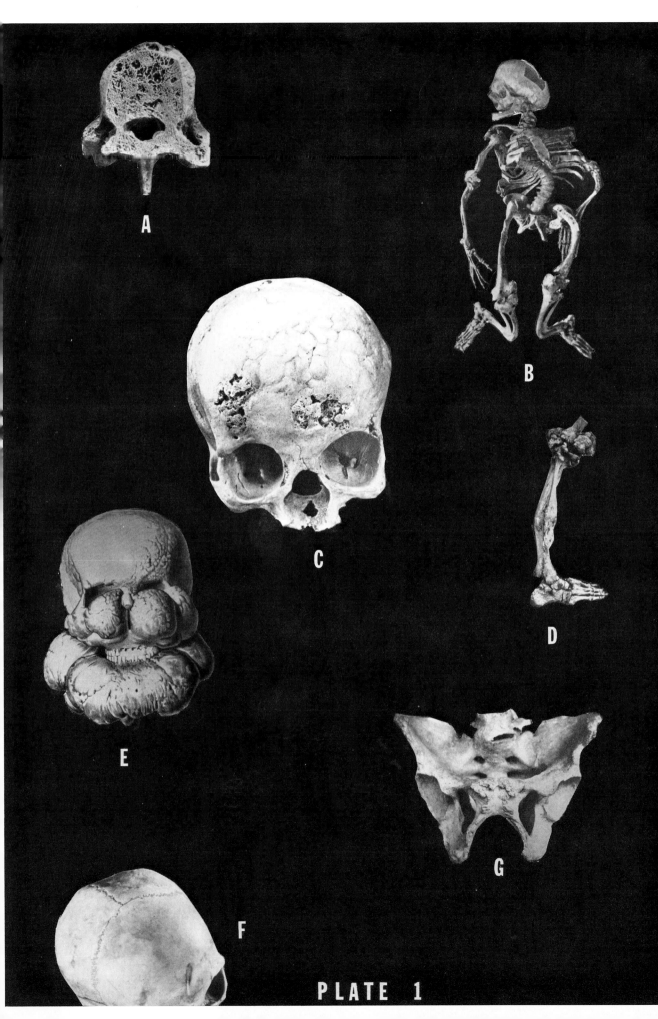

PLATE 1

PLATE 2

DOCUMENTED BONE PATHOLOGY

CIVIL WAR WOUNDS

A. Two round balls caused comminuted fracture, lower left femur. Wounded May 3, 1863. Leg amputated May 10, 1863. Duration 7 days. Bone fragments are sharp. No evidence of bone regeneration or resorption. Specimen No. 1076. (Otis and Huntington, *Medical and Surgical History of the War of the Rebellion*, Part III, Vol. II, Plate XLII.)

B. Gunshot fracture of left ilium. Wounded April 6, 1865. Died April 28, 1865. Duration 22 days. No noticeable bone changes. Specimen No. 4130. (*Ibid.*, Part II, Vol. II, Plate XXXV.)

C. Penetration wound of right hip. The ball went through upper right ilium. Complicated by purulent abscess which ruptured into the abdominal cavity. Wounded July 9, 1864. Died Sept. 10, 1864. Duration 2 months. Photograph shows some minor bone regeneration with roughening and resorption. Specimen No. 3900. (*Ibid.*, Part II, Vol. II, Plate XXXIV.)

D. Gunshot wound left forearm. Complicated by hemorrhage and suppuration. Wounded July 11, 1864. Amputated Feb. 15, 1865. Duration 7 months. Necrosis. Sequestrum (removed from stump at a later date) and extensive involucra. Specimen Nos. 3686 and 3727. (*Ibid.*, Part II, Vol. II, Plate XLVIII.)

E. Gunshot wound. Right elbow with compound fracture lower portion of humerus. Complication, purulent infection. Wounded May 5, 1862. Died August 20, 1863. Duration 15 months. Regeneration of bone, destruction and sequestrum formation. Specimen No. 2749. (*Ibid.*, Part II, Vol. II, Plate XIX.)

F. Severe wound right thigh by a minie ball causing comminuted fracture of femur. Was splinted and healing occurred. Patient able to walk without crutch or cane. Wounded Sept. 19, 1864. Died March 6, 1876. Duration 12 years. Cause of death probably not related to wound. The photograph shows two views of right femur. Appears well healed. Specimen No. 6596. (*Ibid.*, Part III, Vol. II, Plate LV.)

Note: All specimens from Surgical Section, Army Medical Museum.

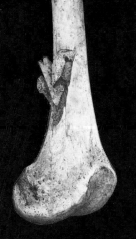

A 7 Days

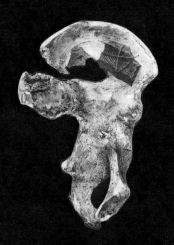

B 22 Days

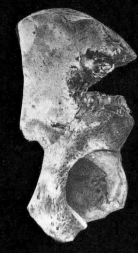

C 2 Months

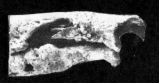

W a r

W o u n d s

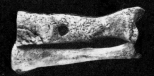

D 7 Months

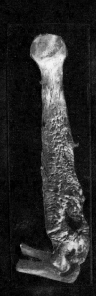

E 15 Months

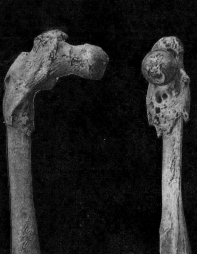

F 12 Years

PLATE 2

PLATE 3

PREHISTORIC FRACTURES

A. Well-healed fracture upper third left femur. Burial No. 29, Male, age 47, buried with child. *In situ*, Emmons Site, Fulton Co., Ill. Mississippian Culture.

B. Posterior view of both femora of A, demonstrating no deformity.

C. Fracture midportion right humerus. Slight rotation and angulation. Female, age 41 to 46. Steuben Site, Marshall Co., Ill. Late Hopewell Culture. Dickson Mounds Collection.

D. Fracture right humerus (posterior view). Healed "Greenstick" (?). Crable Site, Fulton Co., Ill. Mississippian Culture. Dickson Mounds Collection.

E. Compression fracture of second lumbar vertebra. Burial No. 267, Male, age 30. Dickson Mound (F34), Fulton Co., Ill. Mississippian Culture.

F. X-ray of E, demonstrating bony bridging which acted as splints, resulting in complete healing.

G. Fracture right side nasal bone, healing at time of death. Burial No. 95, Female, age 31. Klunk Site (C40), Calhoun Co., Ill. Hopewell Culture. Gilcrease Foundation Collection. Excavated by Gregory Perino.

H. Healed fracture proximal third of right femur with slightly unusual angulation. Burial No. 7, Male, age 26. Morse Site (F772), Fulton Co., Ill. Red Ocher Culture (Late Archaic).

I. Healed fracture, distal ends of left tibia and fibula. Burial No. 20, Male, age 46. Klunk Site (C30), Calhoun Co., Ill. Hopewell Culture. Gilcrease Foundation Collection.

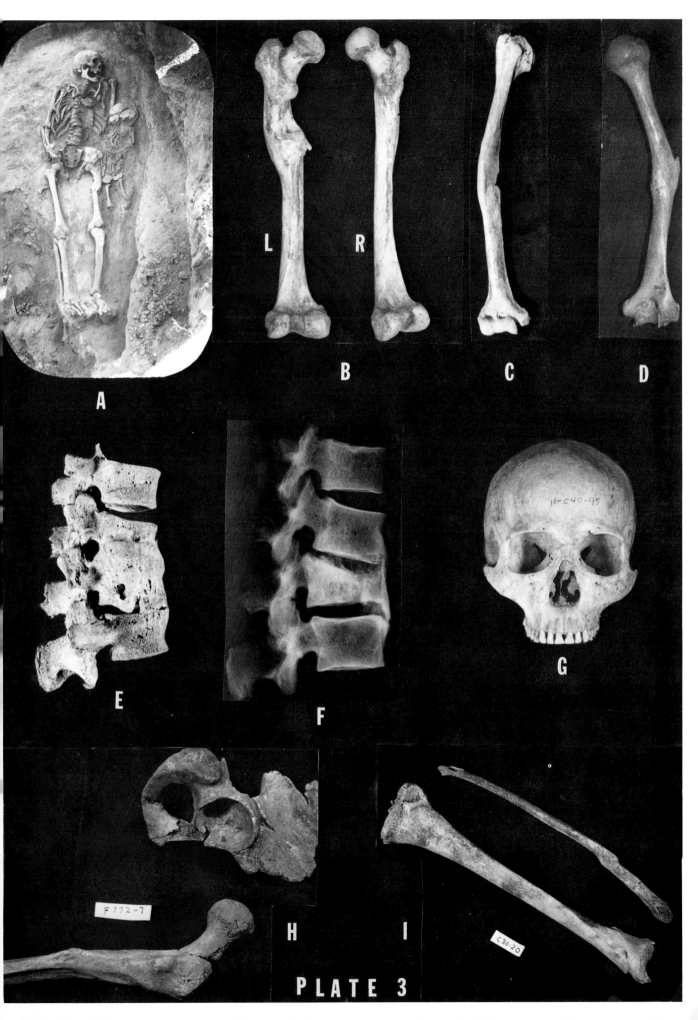

PLATE 3

PLATE 4

PREHISTORIC FRACTURES

Six fractures in one individual. Vandeventer Site, Brown Co., Ill. Mississippian Culture. Dickson Mounds Collection. Excavated by Charles Harris.

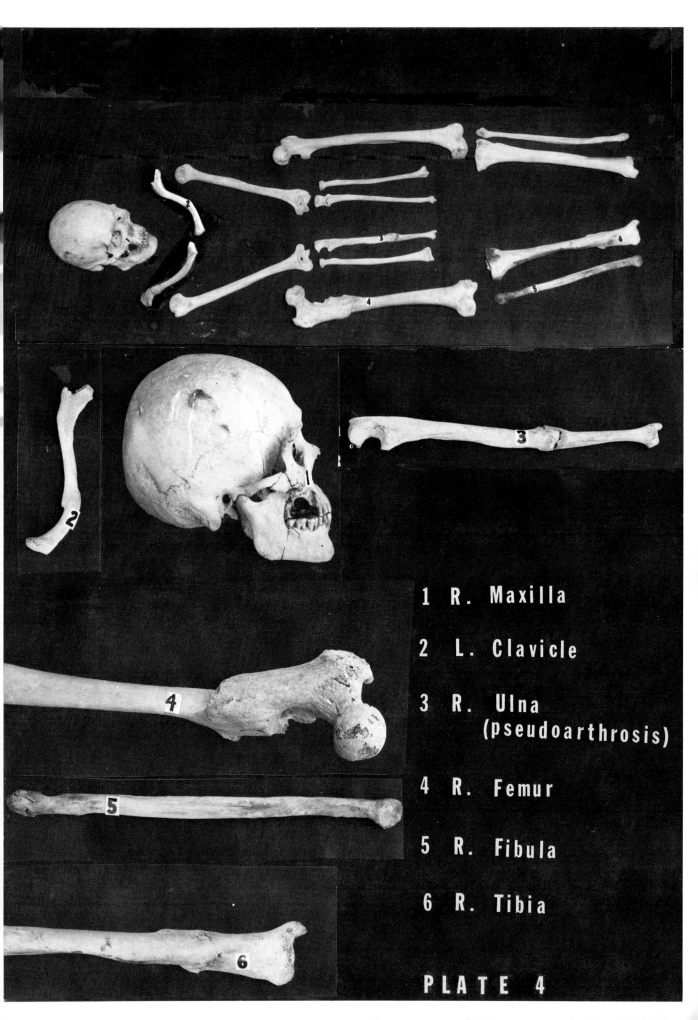

1 R. Maxilla

2 L. Clavicle

3 R. Ulna
  (pseudoarthrosis)

4 R. Femur

5 R. Fibula

6 R. Tibia

PLATE 4

PLATE 5

PREHISTORIC ARROW WOUNDS

A. Arrow point in body of 8th thoracic vertebra. No healing. It is not likely that this arrow wound could have been the cause of death. Female, age 28. Emmons Cemetery, Fulton Co., Ill. Mississippian Culture.

B. Lumbar vertebra found with many other reburied bones. The arrow must have penetrated the spinal cord. Crable Site, Fulton Co., Ill. Mississippian Culture. Found by Marion Dickson.

C. Small Woodland-type arrow imbedded near right occipital condyle. The first cervical vertebra is congenitally fused to occipital bone (unrelated to injury). Adult Male. Indian Mound Park, Adams Co., Ill. Late Woodland Culture.

D. Lower thoracic vertebra. Small triangular Mississippian arrow imbedded in anterior vertebral body. Projectile point must have entered anterior part of body, either chest or abdomen. Dickson Mound (F34), Fulton Co., Ill., prior to systematic excavations. Mississippian Culture.

E. Arrow fragment, broken on both ends, in a lumbar vertebra. Spinal canal was penetrated. Frederick Site, Schuyler Co., Ill. Probably Hopewell Culture. Found by Rod Hiles and Marion Dickson.

F. Late Woodland stemmed arrowpoint penetrating right neural arch of fifth lumbar vertebra. No evidence of healing. Cord injury and immediate death is most likely. Burial 3, Male, age 46. Klunk Site (C34), Calhoun Co., Ill. Hopewell Culture. Gilcrease Foundation Collection. Excavated by Gregory Perino.

G. Child with arrow imbedded in sacrum. Dickson Mound (F34), Fulton Co., Ill., found prior to systematic excavations. Mississippian Culture.

H. Mississippian arrow in two pieces close together lying in upper left thoracic cavity. No damage to bones found. Burial No. 287, Male, age 30. *In situ*, Dickson Mound (F34), Fulton Co., Ill. Mississippian Culture.

I. Arrow, 22 mm. in length, penetrated upper right sacrum. This wound caused death or occurred at time of death. Female, age 47. Klunk Site, Calhoun Co., Ill. Late Woodland Culture. Excavated by Gregory Perino.

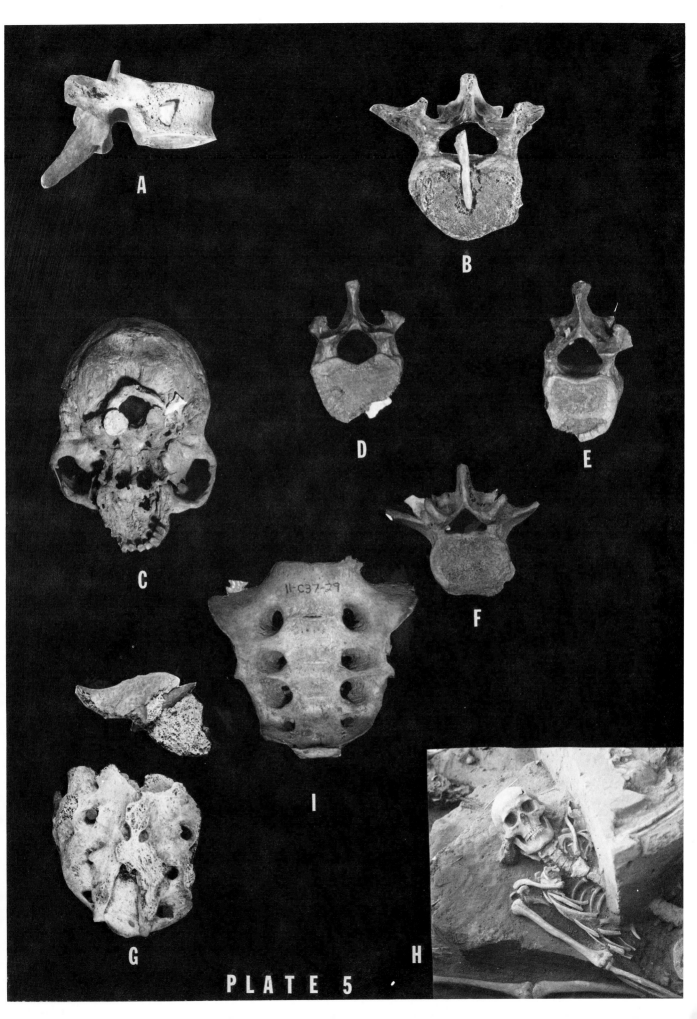

PLATE 5

PLATE 6

PREHISTORIC TRAUMA

A. Unreduced dislocation of right hip. Right acetabulum is shallow and distorted with slight roughening of the surface and shows no evidence of articulation with head of femur. On the anterior surface of the ilium is a shallow false facet which shows evidence of articulation with the deformed head of femur. The right leg would be shortened with an inward angulation. Burial No. 277, female. Dickson Mound (F34), Fulton Co., Ill. Mississippian Culture.

B. A partial burial of a child about 10 years of age showing bilateral congenital dislocation of the hip joints. The left acetabulum is shallow with roughened surfaces. The right inominate is missing. There is pronounced atrophy of the heads of both femora. Burial No. 10, Morse Site (F707), Fulton Co., Ill. Red Ocher Culture (Late Archaic).

C & D. Possible amputation of right hand (healed). Distal ends of radius and ulna fused with a rounded enlargement on distal end of radius. Trauma may be the cause instead of surgery. Burial No. 51, Male, age 42. Klunk Site (C36), Calhoun Co., Ill. Hopewell Culture. Found by Gregory Perino.

E. The knees are flexed in the grave (the only burial in the mound so positioned). There is minimal lipping at the ends of almost all the long bones, including the metacarpals, and lipping of all vertebrae, most severe in the lumbar region. This may be a case of rheumatoid arthritis where there is severe deformity without marked bone disease (See chapter on arthritis). Burial No. 48, Male, age 75. *In situ*, Dickson Mound (F34), Fulton Co., Ill. Mississippian Culture.

F. Close-up of the left foot of E illustrating the result of a crushing injury totally unrelated to the arthritis. The left tibia and fibula are fused together at their distal ends and to all the tarsal bones, making one bony mass with bone boundaries not distinguishable. All metatarsals are distinct except the second which shows evidence of partial bone fusion.

G. The right clavicle is thickened and there is a raised facet (2 x 1.5 cm.) located at the site of the conoid and trapezoid ligaments. There is a very faintly outlined indefinite facet at the superior anterior surface of the coracoid process of the scapula. The right humerus is thickened as a result of fracture or trauma. This is undoubtedly a traumatic lesion with possible shoulder dislocation or an acromioclavicular separation. This same individual had a healed fracture of the spine (See Plate 3,E,F). Burial No. 267, Male, age 30. Dickson Mound (F34), Fulton Co., Ill. Mississippian Culture.

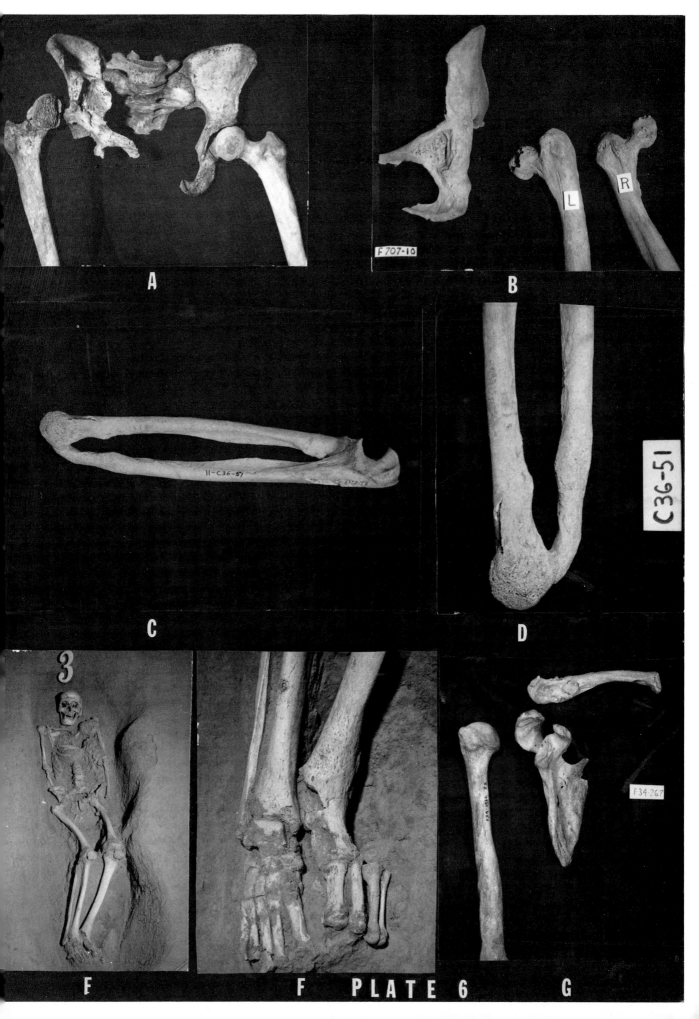

A

B

F707-10

L R

C

11-C36-51

D

C36-51

3

F

F

PLATE 6

G

F34-267

PLATE 7

PREHISTORIC SKULL DEFECTS

A. Three adult males in one burial pit; the upper one (Burial No. 29) has a hole in the skull. Closeup views show complete healing. Morse Site, (F772), Fulton Co., Ill. Red Ocher Culture (Late Archaic). Indiana University Collection. *Closeup photograph, courtesy Illinois State Museum.*

B. Well-healed gash in left frontal region. Adult male. Bear Creek Area, Adams Co., Ill. Late Woodland Culture. Collection of Dr. James Reed, Quincy, Illinois.

C. Skull described by Dr. Georg Neumann as exhibiting evidence of prehistoric scalping (See text). Crable Site, Fulton Co., Ill. Mississippian Culture.

D. An irregularly shaped hole, 5 cm. long, on the left side of frontal bone demonstrating healing along beveled edges. Burial No. 106, Male, age 40. *In situ*, Dickson Mound (F34), Fulton Co., Ill. Mississippian Culture.

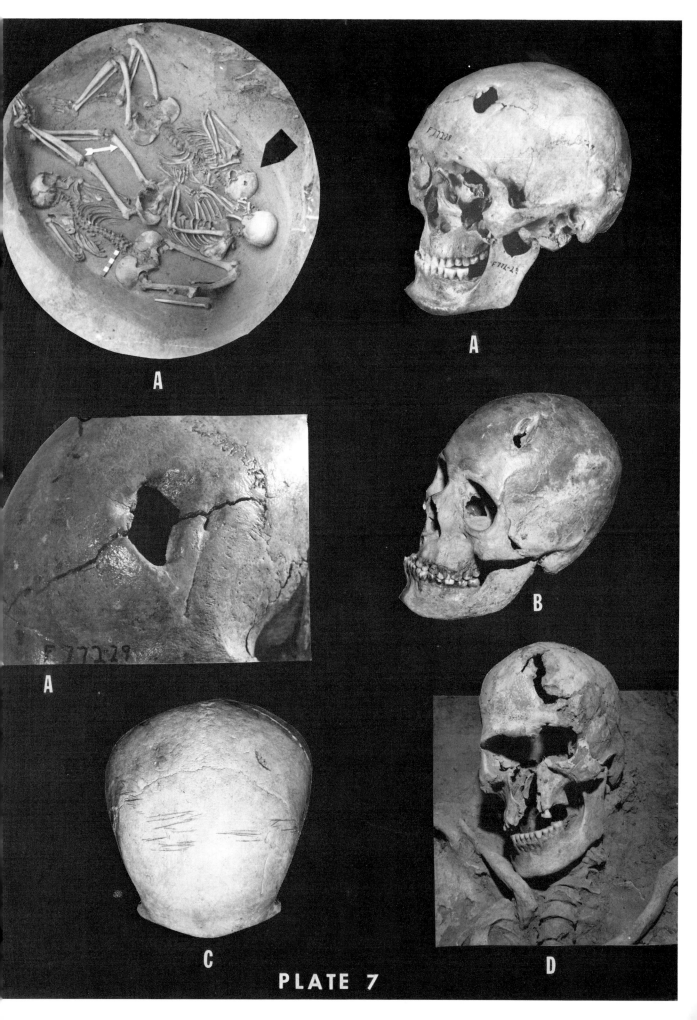

A

A

B

A

C

D

PLATE 7

PLATE 8

PREHISTORIC SKULL DEFECTS

A. Reported as "trephination," it is probably a postmortem perforation with smoothed and polished edges. The surrounding bone shows no evidence of regeneration or bone reaction of any kind. The hole, a little under 2 cm. in diameter, is nearly a perfect circle. The edges are straight. Found in a mound in 1875 by the Rev. Dr. Pilcher, near Devil River, Michigan (Hinsdale and Greenman 1936). Museum of Anthropology Collection, University of Michigan.

B. An oblong-shaped bone defect (4 x 2.5 cm.) located at the junction of the sagittal and coronal sutures. The edges are straight or slanting. The bone wound is well healed. There is some minor pitting surrounding the hole. This is a possible trephinization, but trauma cannot be ruled out. A surgical approach in this location shows lack of judgment and/or experience as surgery would likely open up the large venous sinuses. Blue Creek Site, Pike Co.. Ill. Hopewell Culture. (McGregor and Wadlow 1951)

C. This is most likely a spear or knife wound. There is no evidence of healing. Dickson Mound (F34), Fulton Co., Ill. Mississippian Culture.

D. Reported as a trephinization because of the square-shaped hole and some evidence of prolongation of cuts. Unfortunately only the top of the skull was found. If the specimen were more complete, one might be more certain that this was surgery and not trauma. Evidence of healing is unconvincing. Ethel H. Wilson Site (WH7), White Co., Ill. Hopewell Culture. (Neumann and Fowler 1952:211)

E. Skull showing two holes. The lower one was well healed; the upper and larger defect shows minor evidence of bone regeneration of the edges. Riviere aux Vase Site, Macomb Co., Mich. Museum of Anthropology Collection, University of Michigan.

F. A skull with a circular hole. The edges are slanting and indicate complete healing. Trauma is the most likely cause. Beckstead Site, Fulton Co., Ill. Mississippian Culture, Dickson Mounds Collection.

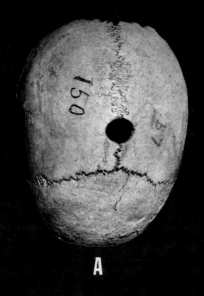

A

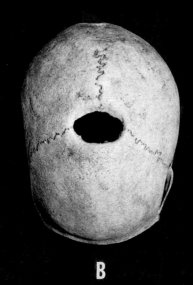

B

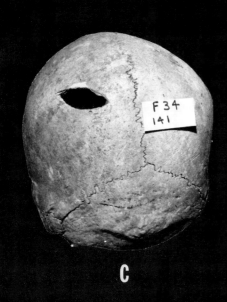

C

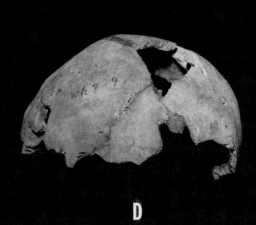

D

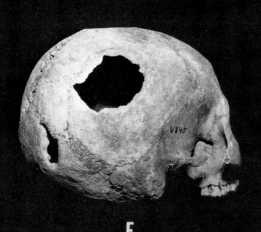

E

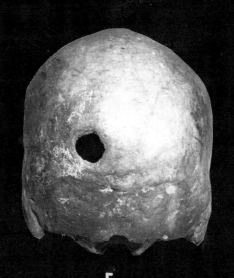

F

PLATE 8

PLATE 9

PERUVIAN TREPHINING

A.   Squier's Skull from Cuzco, Peru. Crosshatched cuts. Pictured in many books (Moodie 1923; Stewart 1958; and others).

B.   Skull from Cuzco with seven trephined openings in various degrees of healing (Oakley et al 1959).

C.   Child, age about six. Rectangular hole (Stewart 1958, Plate 9).

D.   Angular area of osteitis surrounding opening. U. S. National Museum. (Stewart 1966:44).

E.   Hole made by multiple drilling (rare). (Drawn from photograph in Moodie's *Paleopathology*, 1923. Plate CIX.)

Drawings by Alan Harn.

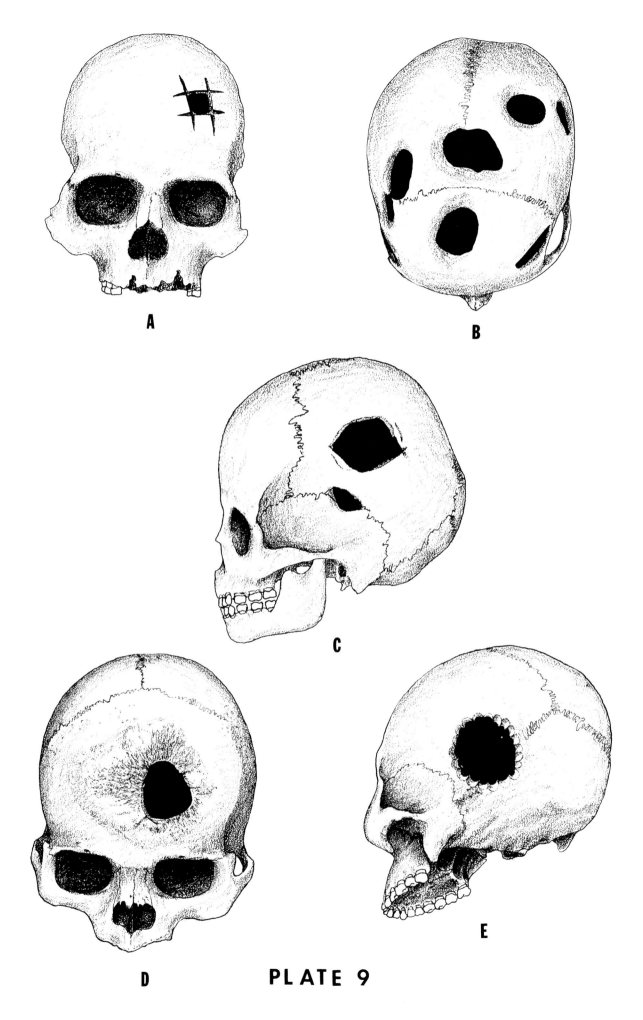

A

B

C

D

E

PLATE 9

PLATE 10

PREHISTORIC TRAUMA

A. Scarifier, consisting of eight small pointed bone needles, located just above the left shoulder. Burial No. 12, Male, age 40. Emmons Cemetery, Fulton Co., Ill. Mississippian Culture.

B. Deformity at the proximal end of the first metacarpal bone (Bennett's Fracture). X-ray of left and right first metacarpals. Male, age 63. Schild Site, Green Co., Ill. Early Mississippian Culture. Excavated by Gregory Perino.

C. Greatly thickened right tibia. The bone was sawed through longitudinally. The sawing was very difficult because of increased bone density, most likely a reaction to trauma. This was a bundle burial. No other bones were abnormal. Burial No. 56, Male, over 50 years of age. Steuben Site, Mound 1, Marshall Co., Ill. Hopewell Culture. (Dan F. Morse 1963:94)

D. Microscopic sections of C, showing a marked increase in the density of cortical bone.

E. Localized osteosclerotic bulging of anterior medial surface of middle portion of right tibia (arrow). This is undoubtedly a local reaction to trauma, with or without a fracture. Left tibia is shown for comparison. Burial No. 34, Female, over 50 years of age. Klunk Site (C31), Calhoun Co., Ill. Hopewell Culture.

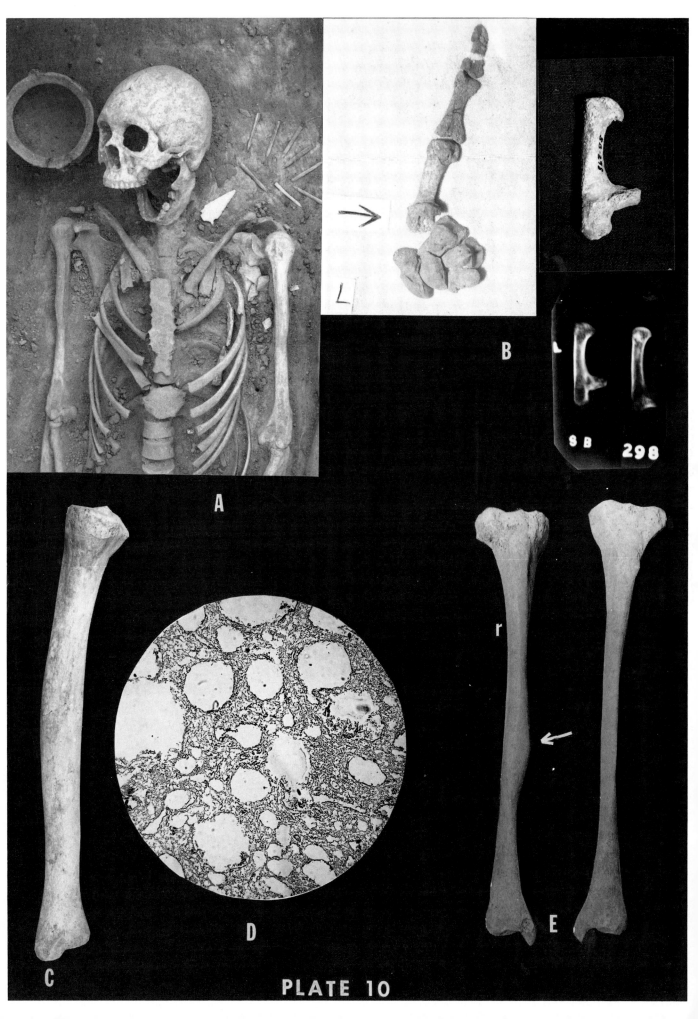

PLATE 10

PLATE 11

ARTHRITIS

A. Rheumatoid arthritis. Lipping and minimal erosion of the bone ends is present on nearly all the joints including those of the hands and feet. The fusion of the left foot bones is a separate entity not related to the arthritis. Burial No. 48. Dickson Mound (F34), Fulton Co., Ill. Mississippian Culture. (See Plate 6,E).

B. X-ray of a spine showing ankylosing spondylitis. Crable Site, Fulton Co., Ill. Mississippian Culture.

C. Severe ankylosing spondylitis involving all vertebrae, sacroiliac, and all costovertebral joints. Burial No. 4, Male, age 47 to 50. Klunk Site (C36), Calhoun Co., Ill. Hopewell Culture.

D. Fusion of pubic bones with pronounced nodule formation. The pelvic opening is diminished in size. Both sacroiliac joints are fused and there is also a fusion of the second and third lumbar vertebrae. Probably a mild or a beginning ankylosing spondylitis (See also Plate 1,G). Burial No. 58, Female, age 34. *In situ*, Dickson Mound (F34), Fulton Co., Ill. Mississippian Culture.

E. Infectious arthritis of the right hip joint; acetabulum shallow and enlarged in circumference; head of the femur grossly deformed and pointed. Two small circular pieces of bone fit into the acetabulum and are probably sequestra from the head of the femur. Burial No. 64. Male, age 57. Klunk Site (C40), Calhoun Co., Ill. Hopewell Culture.

F. Plantar view of the great left toe. There is a fusion of the interphalangeal joint. The surface of the bone is roughened and shows evidence of considerable bony degeneration. Probably infectious arthritis with complete healing. Burial No. 366, Female, age 60. Dickson Mound (F34), Fulton Co., Ill. 1966 excavation. Mississippian Culture.

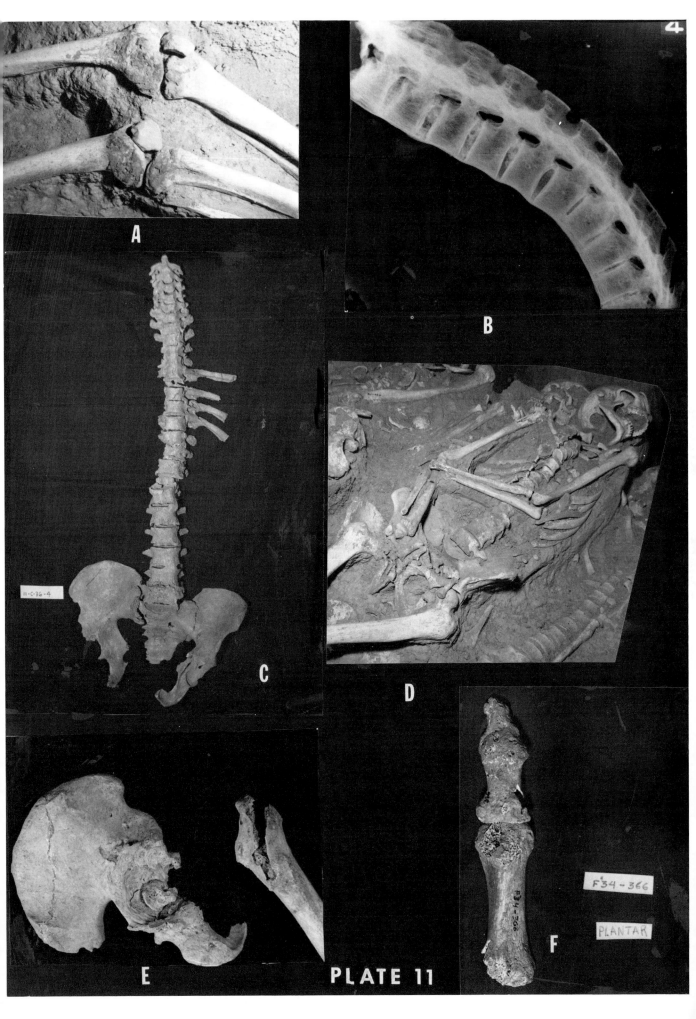

PLATE 11

PLATE 12

ARTHRITIS

A. Right elbow showing traumatic arthritis. Dislocation of the right elbow associated with a fracture of the neck of the radius with reduction resulting in pronounced degenerative changes. There is eburnation of the lateral condylar articular surface of the humerus with marked marginal osteophyte formation. The articular surface of the ulna shows pronounced marginal bony proliferation. The head of the radius is grossly distorted and angulated 45° as a result of a healed fracture of the neck of the radius, resulting in considerable limitation of motion (55° in flexion to 145° in extension). No other joints of this burial show any abnormality. Burial No. 20, Female, age 54. Klunk Site (C37), Calhoun Co., Ill. Late Woodland Culture.

B. Generalized severe arthritis. Left knee illustrated here shows severe lipping and pronounced eburnation of the medial condyles of the femur and tibia. Burial No. 32, Male, age 64. Klunk Site (C37), Calhoun Co., Ill. Late Woodland Culture.

C. The left knee exhibits pronounced degenerative changes. There is lipping of the margins of the joint and erosion of the articular borders. A bony spur at the distal end of the patella seriously interfered with the motion of the knee joint. All the joints of this burial were involved in a moderate to severe arthritis. Male, age 63. Schild Site, Green Co., Ill. Mississippian Culture.

D. Osteoarthritis involving bones of feet, principally the metatarsals and phalanges. Burial No. 245, Adult, sex not determined. Dickson Mound (F34), Fulton Co., Ill. Mississippian Culture.

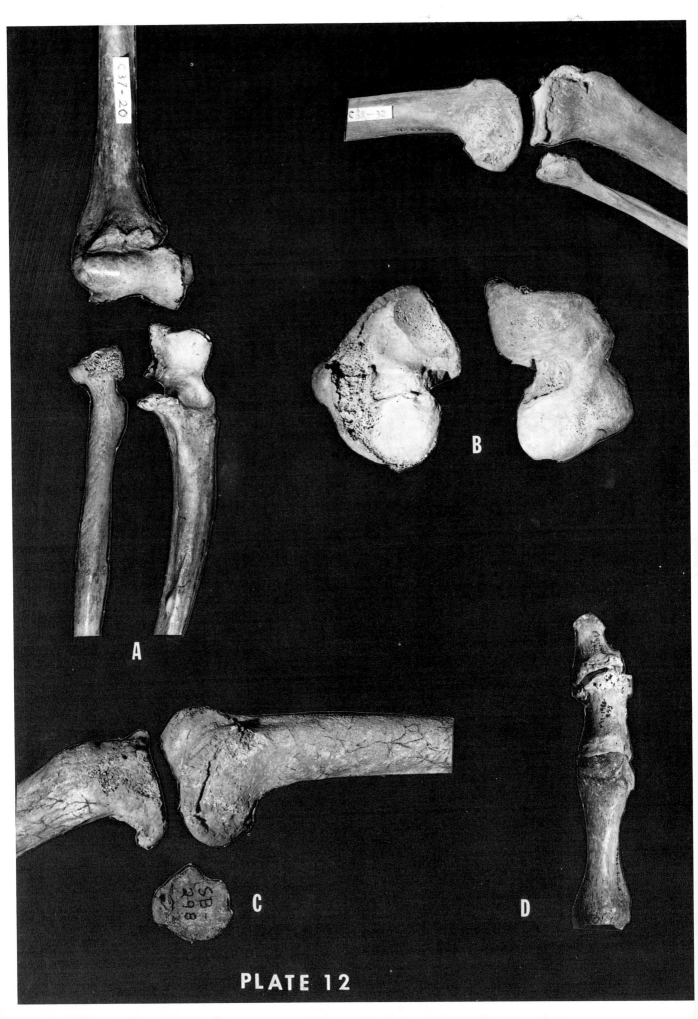

PLATE 12

PLATE 13

PERIOSTITIS

A. Pronounced periostitis located, for the most part, on the anterior surfaces of the femora, tibiae, and fibulae. Periostitis also evident on the anterior surfaces of the second through fifth lumbar vertebrae, the distal end of the left humerus, one rib fragment, and a moderate amount on the sacrum. The skull is not affected. Burial No. 12, Female, age 22. Morse Site (F772), Fulton Co., Ill. Red Ocher Culture (Late Archaic).

B. Closeup view of proximal end of left tibia of A.

C. This burial shows a generalized periostitis involving parts of the clavicles, left humerus, left ulna, both fibulae, right scapula, and anterior surface of left tibia. The skull is normal. Closeup view, anterior surface of left tibia. Burial No. 42, Male, age 48. Klunk Site (C34), Calhoun Co., Ill. Hopewell Culture.

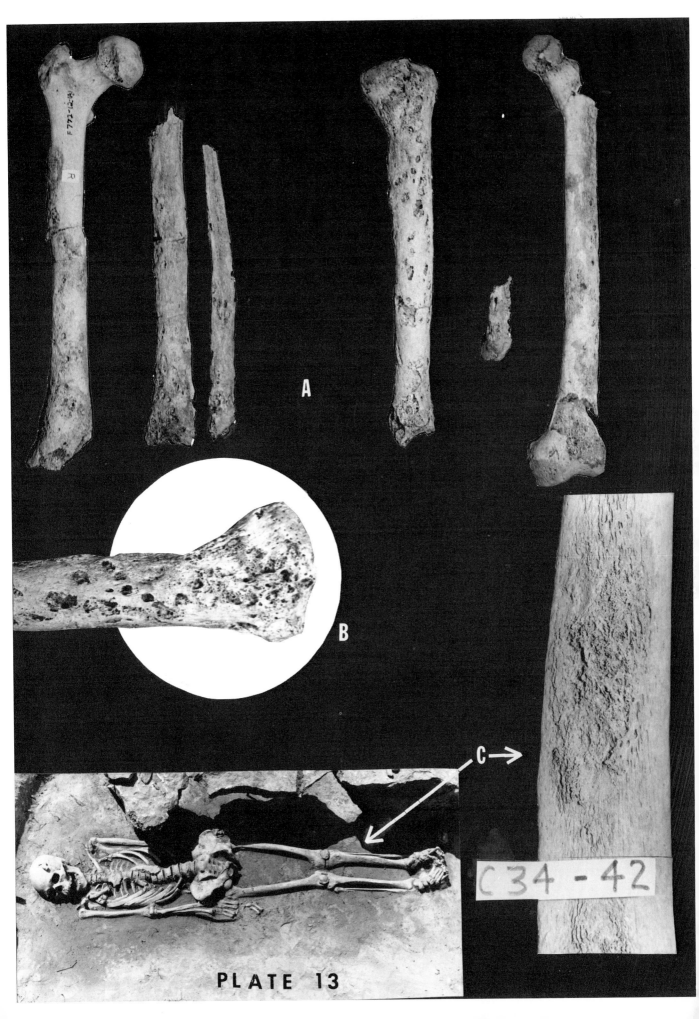

A

B

C→

C34-42

PLATE 13

PLATE 14

PERIOSTITIS

A. Severe periostitis and osteitis over anterior portion of frontal bone. The disease is not healed and was active at time of death. Burial No. 1, Male, age 26. Klunk Site (C30), Calhoun Co., Ill. Hopewell Culture.

B. The entire right tibia was involved in severe periostitis characterized by irregular surfaces eroded by many irregularly shaped pits, from tiny to 5 mm. in diameter and 1 to 2 mm. in depth. The left tibia grossly appears normal, but x-ray shows mild periostitis located in the proximal third. Burial No. 284, (Note: Burial No. was changed from F°34-1966-52 to F°34-284.), Female, age 38. Dickson Mound (F34), Fulton Co., Ill. Mississippian Culture.

C. Distal ends of the left tibia and fibula showing many osteophytes projecting distally. There is a generalized periostitis involving most of the long bones as evidenced by roughened surfaces with periosteal erosion and some cortical thickening. The skull is normal. Burial No. 41, Male, age 35. Klunk Site (C31), Calhoun Co., Ill. Hopewell Culture.

D. Periostitis of all surfaces of both tibia. No other bone involvement. Burial No. 40, Female, age 35. Klunk Site (C36), Calhoun Co., Ill. Hopewell Culture.

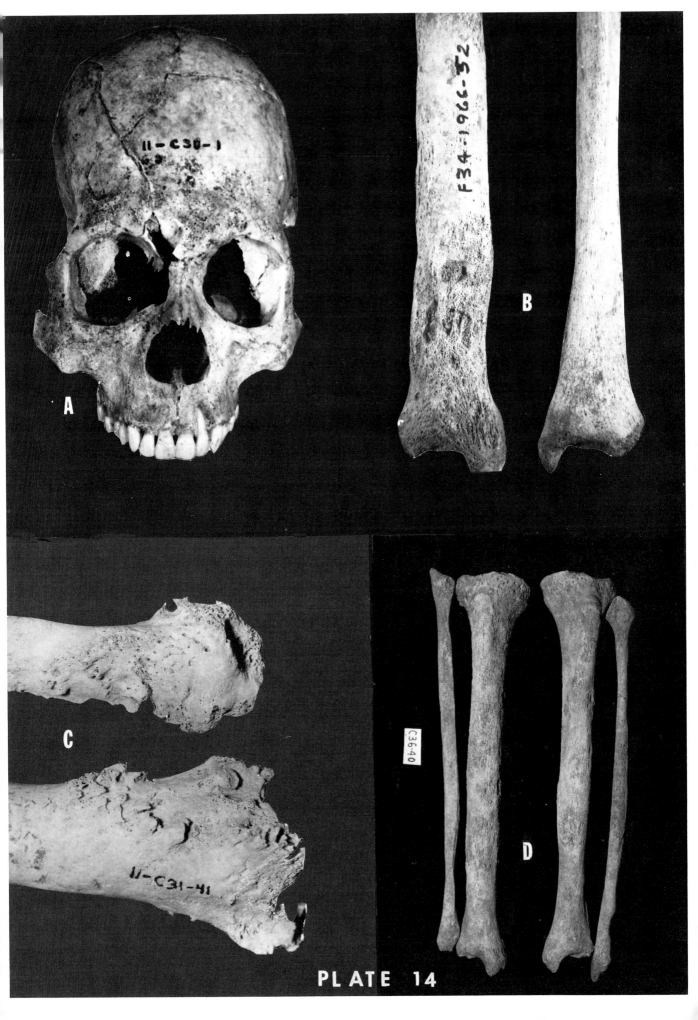

PLATE 14

PLATE 15

PERIOSTITIS

A-C: This individual may have had a severe treponema infection, re-
sulting in death, or some obscure metabolic disease or anemia.
Burial No. 21, Male, age 41. Klunk Site (C40), Calhoun Co., Ill.
Hopewell Culture.

A. The skull has some longitudinal bulges of new bone with many
holes and pits over most of the cranial surface. The bone appears
to be thickened, becoming quite thin near the holes.

B. There is periostitis over the surfaces of most of the long bones.
The surfaces are covered with many small irregular pits, ranging
from $\frac{1}{2}$ mm. to 5 mm. in diameter, between which are tiny trabeculae of new bone. This process is scattered over the surfaces of
both tibiae, both femora, distal ends of both humeri (mild), midportion right radius, distal end of left radius, midportion right
ulna, proximal end of left ulna, and scattered over both fibulae.
There is no involvement of fingers, toes, ribs, or vertebrae. No
joint surfaces are involved.

C. The marrow spaces are obliterated in the right tibiae, both fibulae,
both ulnae and the right clavicle. The condition of the marrow
spaces was not determined in the left tibia, left clavicle, and left
femur because there were no breaks. The marrow spaces are present but decreased in the right femur and upper end of the radius.
X-rays and microscopic sections have eliminated Paget's disease.

D-F: In addition to the cranial involvement, this burial shows a swelling of the upper third of the left tibia, the surface of which is
irregular and demonstrates a periosteal reaction. Burial No. 294
(bundle burial), Female, age 36. Dickson Mound (F34), Fulton
Co., Ill. Mississippian Culture.

D. There are two holes in the skull. The first hole, 1 cm. in diameter,
is located in the midsagittal suture.

E. The second, located in the mid-right parietal bone, measures 1 cm.
in diameter. It is circular in shape.

F. Pitting on the interior surface demonstrates that the lesion probably originated from within.

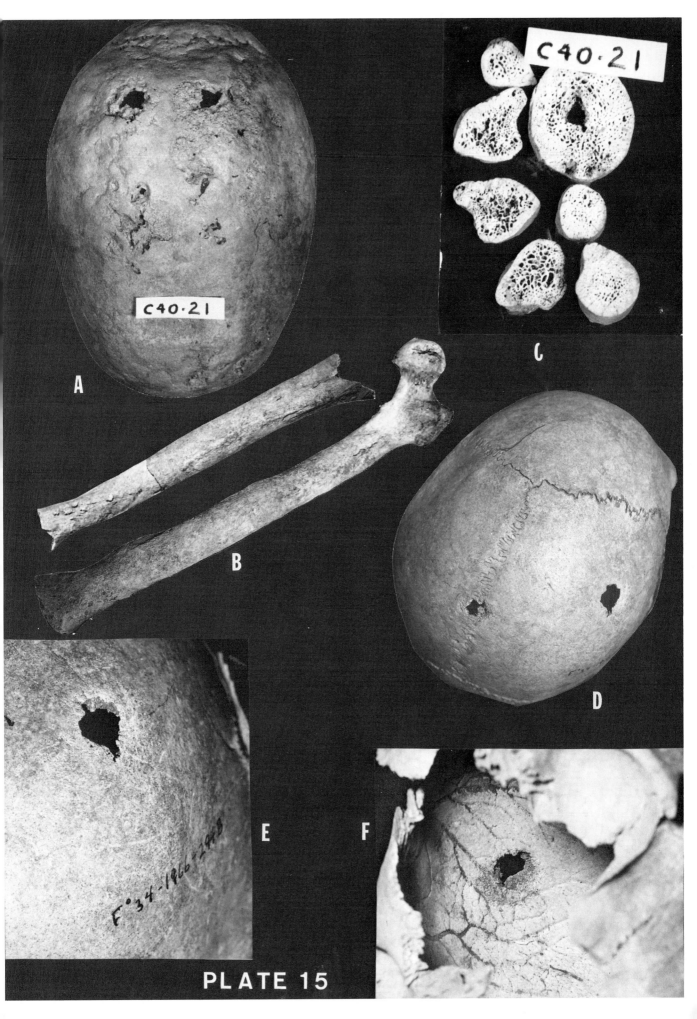

A   C40·21

C

B

D

E   F

PLATE 15

PLATE 16

OSTEOMYELITIS

A. Right and left femur. Right femur is greatly thickened because the entire bone is surrounded by a shell of new bone (involucrum). The x-ray shows original cortex. A′ shows cross section demonstrating that the shaft is a sequestrum surrounded by the involucrum. Burial No. 391, Infant. Dickson Mound (F34), Fulton Co., Ill. Mississippian Culture.

B. Severe destructive osteomyelitis of left tibia and fibula. The rest of the bones were normal. Burial No. 32. Morse Site (F772), Fulton Co., Ill. Red Ocher Culture (Late Archaic).

C. View of right and left femur. The left femur demonstrates a severe osteomyelitis that started before the growth period was completed. It had never completely healed and was still active at time of death. Adult. Crable Site, Fulton Co., Ill. Mississippian Culture.

D. Osteomyelitis of the left portion of occipital bone demonstrating incomplete healing at time of death. Probably initiated by a blow or injury. Adult male. Nutwood Site, Jersey Co., Ill. Bluff Culture (Late Woodland).

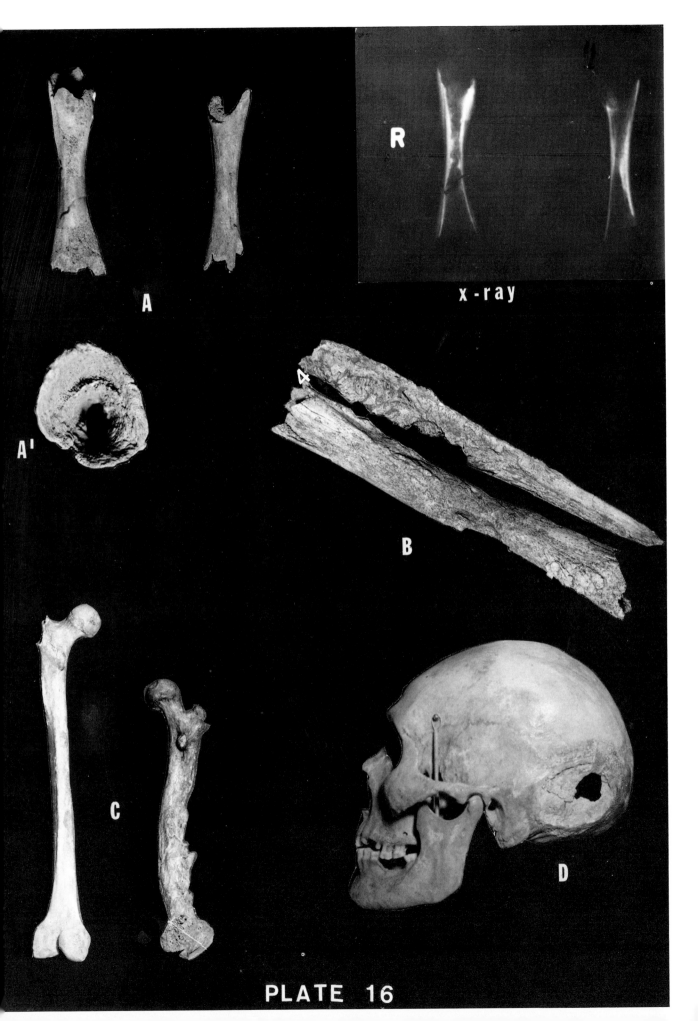

x-ray

A

A'

B

C

D

R

PLATE 16

PLATE 17

OSTEOMYELITIS

A. The skull of the lowest skeleton presents an osteomyelitis probably developing after an injury, resulting in death. The disease in the left femur and right tibia rather closely resembles a non-suppurative chronic osteomyelitis of Garré. Burial No. 293, Male, age 20. Dickson Mound (F34), Fulton Co., Ill. Mississippian Culture.

B. The skull of Burial No. 293 with the sequestrum removed.

C. Periosteal thickening with pitting surrounding the hole in the skull. Burial No. 293.

D. Lower half of left femur showing thickening of the lower third with no sinus tract visible. Burial No. 293.

E. Upper half of the right tibia showing the thickening with a single healed sinus tract. X-ray of the right and left tibia shows considerable cortical thickening and a decrease in the size of the marrow space on the right. Left is normal for comparison. Burial No. 293.

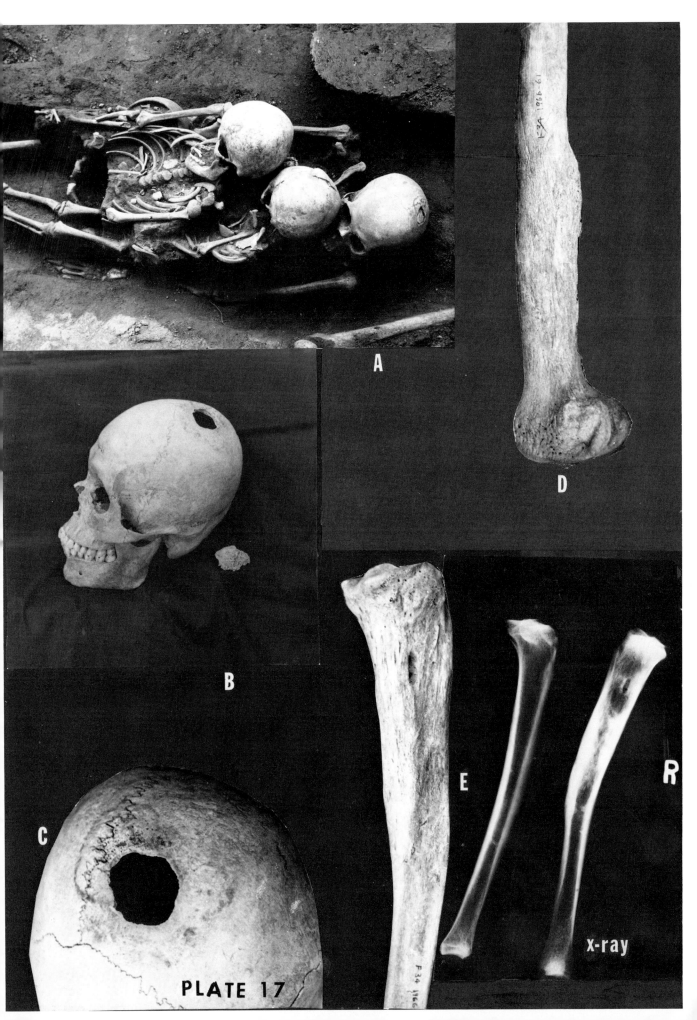

A

B

C

D

E

R

x-ray

PLATE 17

PLATE 18

OSTEOPHYTOSIS AND BONE CYST

A. Mild osteophytosis showing vertebral lipping. Burial No. 12, Female, age 22. Morse Site (F772), Fulton Co., Ill. Red Ocher Culture (Late Archaic).

B. Lumbar vertebral osteophytosis with large bony prominence projecting anteriorly from the body of the fifth lumbar vertebra. Burial No. 17A, Female, age 50. Morse Site (F707), Fulton Co., Ill. Probably Late Woodland Culture.

C. Severe osteophytosis of all lumbar vertebrae. Burial No. 32, Male, age 64. Klunk Site (C37), Calhoun Co., Ill. Late Woodland Culture.

D. Pronounced bilateral ear exostosis. The mastoid processes were stained green probably from copper earspools. Skull found in gravel pit near Shawneetown, Ill. Culture unknown.

E. Circular hole, located in left frontal bone close to the orbit, measures 7 mm. in diameter and about 5 mm. deep. The hole, with smooth walls, includes the left frontal sinus. The edges are very smooth and beveled outward. There is some minimal roughening of surrounding bone. Possibilities are bone cyst, epidermoid cyst, or mucocele. Burial No. 332, Male, age 65. Dickson Mound (F34), Fulton Co., Ill. Mississippian Culture.

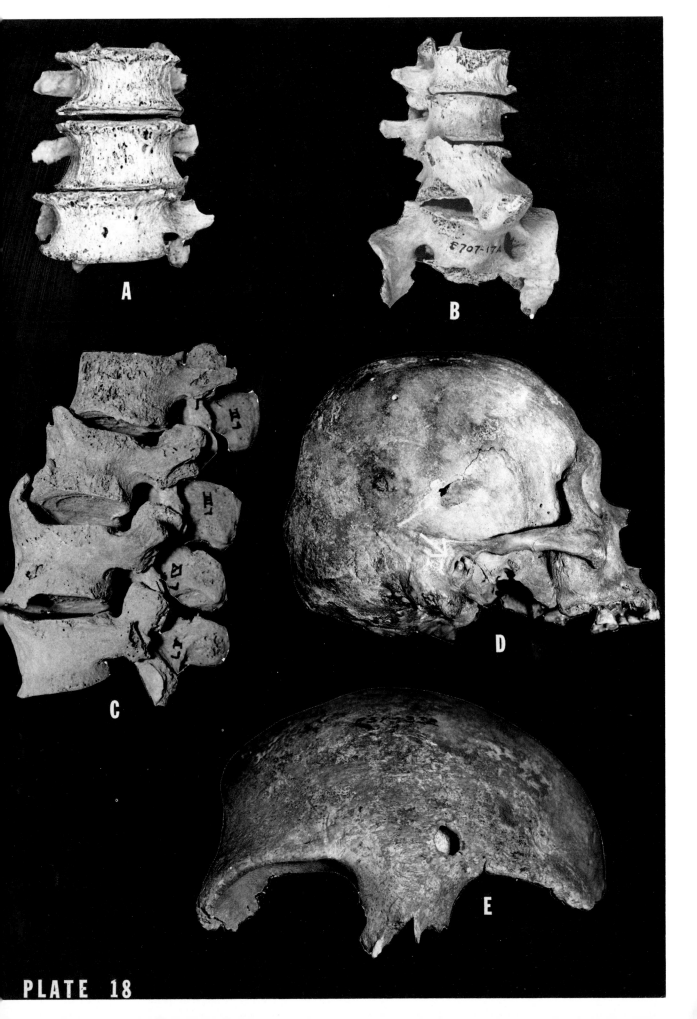

A

B

C

D

E

PLATE 18

PLATE 19

TUMORS

A. Pronounced thickening of right temporal bone. The x-ray shows typical findings of an osteoma. The two cup-like depressions on the frontal bone are probably results of an old injury and have no relationship to the osteoma. Burial No. 16, Male, age 70. Morse Site (F707), Fulton Co., Ill. Late Woodland Culture.

B. Bony spur on the distal end of the left femur. Burial No. 13, Female, age 50. Steuben Site, Mound 1, Marshall Co., Ill. Hopewell Culture.

C. Many bony tumors on anterior surface of right tibia, raised circular plaques with irregular surfaces measuring ½ to 1 cm. in diameter. Probably benign bone tumors. Burial No. 57, Female, age 29. Klunk Site (C40), Calhoun Co., Ill. Hopewell Culture.

D. Several mushroom-shaped raised circular bone papules located on frontal bone, the smallest, 3 mm. in diameter, the largest, 7 mm. It appears that several more were forming. The impression is that these are benign osteomata. Burial No. 72A, Male, age 68. Klunk Site (C30), Calhoun Co., Ill. Hopewell Culture.

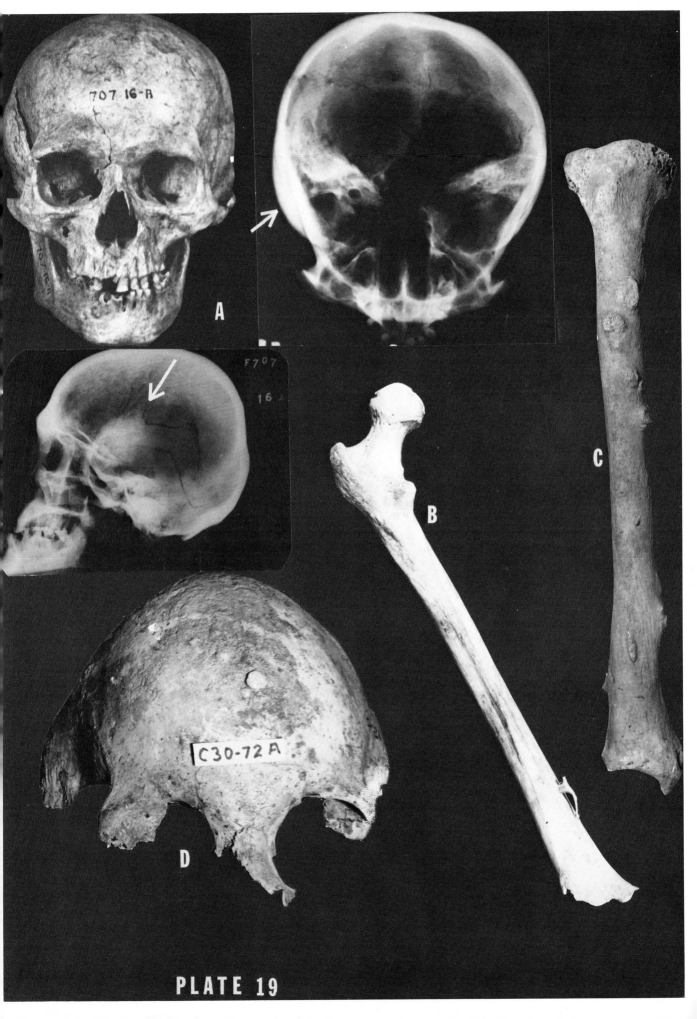

A

B

C

F707 16

707 16-A

C30-72A

D

PLATE 19

PLATE 20

TUMORS

A-B: Burial No. 49, Steuben Site, Mound 1, Marshall Co., Ill. Hopewell Culture.

A.   There is an atrophy of the right side of the lower jaw and of the right zygomatic arch (upper jaw is missing). Unilateral atrophy of the jaw might have been caused by injury to the fifth nerve at its origin or along its course. According to Sarnat and Laskin (1962), asymmetry of the right and left mandible can result when "either one condylar growth center becomes more active than the other, or the growth activity persists in one while the other condyle is no longer active."

B.   In addition there is a deep, rounded depression, about one inch in diameter, located on the internal surface of the skull at the anterior-superior angle of the left parietal bone. The depression is immediately posterior to the coronal suture and lateral to the sagittal suture. Externally a very small prominence, hardly noticeable, is seen directly above the internal depression. Both the internal and external surfaces of this prominence appear intact with no evidence of fracture or bone erosion. The possibilities are a tumor or blood clot on the surface of the brain which pushed the bone outward without causing erosion.

C-D: Burial No. 270, age 2½. Dickson Mound (F34), Fulton Co., Ill. Mississippian Culture.

C.   There is an abscess of the inferior surface of the twelfth thoracic vertebra and the superior surface of the body of the first lumbar vertebra with an opening on its anterior portion. The walls of the abscess are rough and there is no evidence of bone regeneration. It is evident that the cavity or abscess crosses the intervertebral disc.

D.   The left ilium has a multilocular cavity involving its medial posterior surface with evidence of slight trabecular bone regeneration. The auricular facet and the iliac tuberosity are deformed to absent.
     Possible diagnosis: (1) eosinophilic granuloma, (2) tumor, or (3) a low-grade infection. Eosinophilic granuloma would best account for both lesions. Fibrous dysplasia is rare in vertebrae and does not cross the intervertebral disc. Infectious inflammation is not probable because there is very little bone reaction such as one would expect with infection.

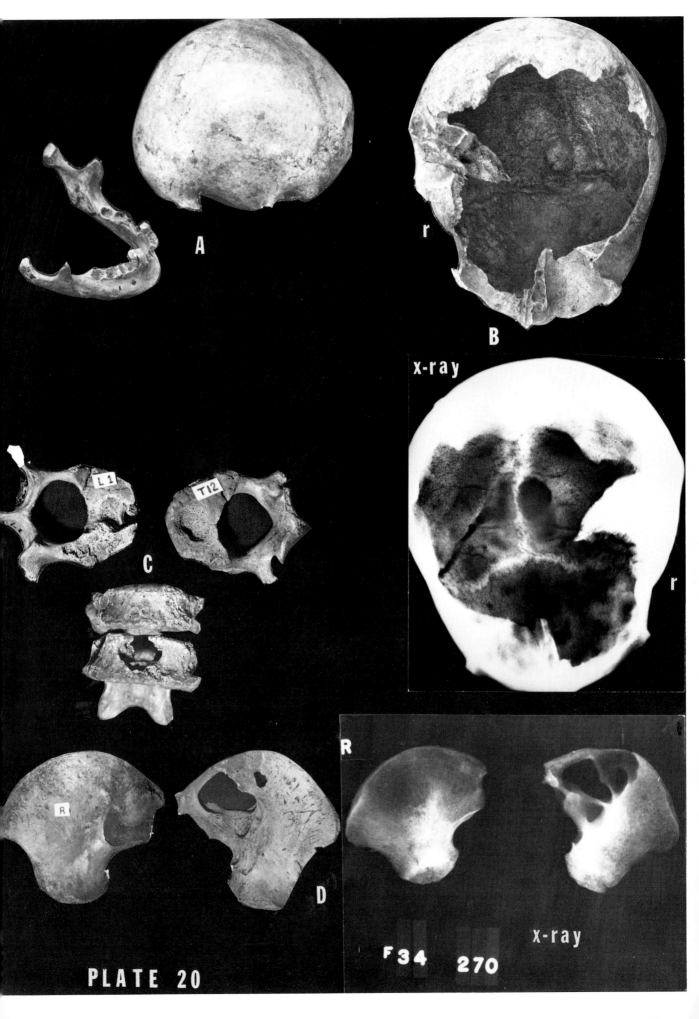

A

B

r

x-ray

r

L 1

T12

C

R

D

R

x-ray

F34 270

PLATE 20

PLATE 21

TUMORS

A. There is a slight bulging of the mid-parietal area. The outer table is intact. X-ray shows an area of rarefaction involving the anterior and superior portion of the parietal with some bone reaction surrounding this area of rarefaction. There is an overgrowth of the inner and outer tables with expansion of the outer table. There is some extension of the process into the adjacent portion of the frontal bone. X-ray reading suggests an erosion of the inner table back of the coronal suture. Examination of the specimen by directing a light so that one can see through the foramen magnum reveals that there is a small break in the inner table but this appears to be due to postmortem changes.

    Diagnosis: Hemangioma is a possibility. The x-ray does show some "honeycombing" but there is no typical "sunray" appearance. Epidermal cyst can be ruled out because the outer table is not perforated. Other more remote possibilities are sarcoma and aneurysmal bone cyst. Dick's Mound, Adams Co., Ill. Late Woodland Culture (ca. A.D. 900).

B. This burial is complete except for the right lower arm and hand. Description of the right humerus: The anatomical neck is normal. The anterior lateral aspect of the proximal metaphysis contains two cavities, one measuring 2 cm. by 1.5 cm. and 1 cm. deep, the other is 1 cm. by 1 cm. and is 1 cm. deep. These cavities extend through the cortex into the marrow space producing condensation of surrounding bone. They are located along the course of the bicipital groove and extend down to the insertion of the pectoralis major muscle. The walls of the cavities are smooth. The diaphysis is grossly normal. A portion of the lower end of the humerus is missing as a result of postmortem changes. That which remains is grossly abnormal with distortion of both condyles and irregularity of the joint surface. The surface is roughened as if it had not been in articulation. On the anterior aspect of the distal metaphysis, just about the articular surface of the medial condyle, is a cavity (similar to those found proximally). This cavity measures 1.3 cm. by 1 cm. and .5 cm. deep. It extends into the medullary space. Its walls are smooth and there is condensation of the surrounding bone.

    Possible diagnosis: (1) Low-grade infection or benign tumor. A benign synovial tumor is most likely and probably originated in the tendon sheaths. The smooth walls would favor tumor rather than infection but it is difficult to account for involvement in both ends of the humerus. (2) Since there was no lower right arm found with this burial and the articular surface of the lower end of the humerus suggests lack of articulation, amputation with survival is probable. Burial No. 451, Male, age 70. Dickson Mound (F34), Fulton Co., Ill. 1967 excavation. Mississippian Culture.

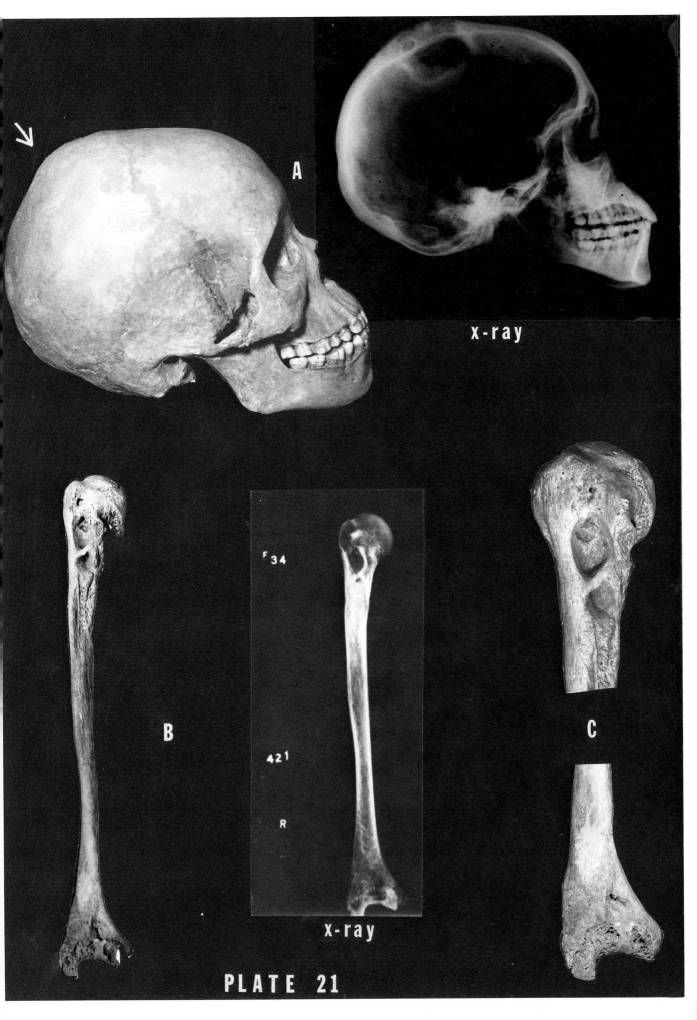

A

x-ray

B

F 34

42 1

R

x-ray

C

PLATE 21

PLATE 22

ANOMALIES

A. There is evidence of atrophy of the bones of the right arm involving the scapula, humerus, radius, and ulna. All bones are shorter and smaller in diameter than those in the left arm. The head of the right humerus is distorted. The cause of this atrophy must be either peripheral or central nerve damage. There may have been an injury to the brachial plexus causing an Erb's palsy. This condition could be caused also by infantile paralysis. Burial No. 39, Male (?), age approximately 15. Klunk Site (C30), Calhoun Co., Ill. Hopewell Culture.

B. Photograph and x-ray of skull from a Late Woodland burial. Most of the burial was in bad condition due to a fire. This individual probably suffered from acromegaly. The long bones which were present were elongated and thickened. The lower jaw is lengthened, the teeth are not materially separated, and the frontal sinuses are not enlarged. Male. Dick's Mound, Adams Co., Ill. (ca. A.D. 900).

C. Spondylolysis of the fifth lumbar vertebra with resulting separation of the spinous process due to a defect in the neural arch. The burial is pictured *in situ* (See Plate 3,A). Male, age 47. Emmons Cemetery, Fulton Co., Ill. Mississippian Culture.

D. Three cases of spondylolysis involving the fifth lumbar vertebra. Morse Site, Fulton Co., Ill. Red Ocher Culture (Late Archaic).

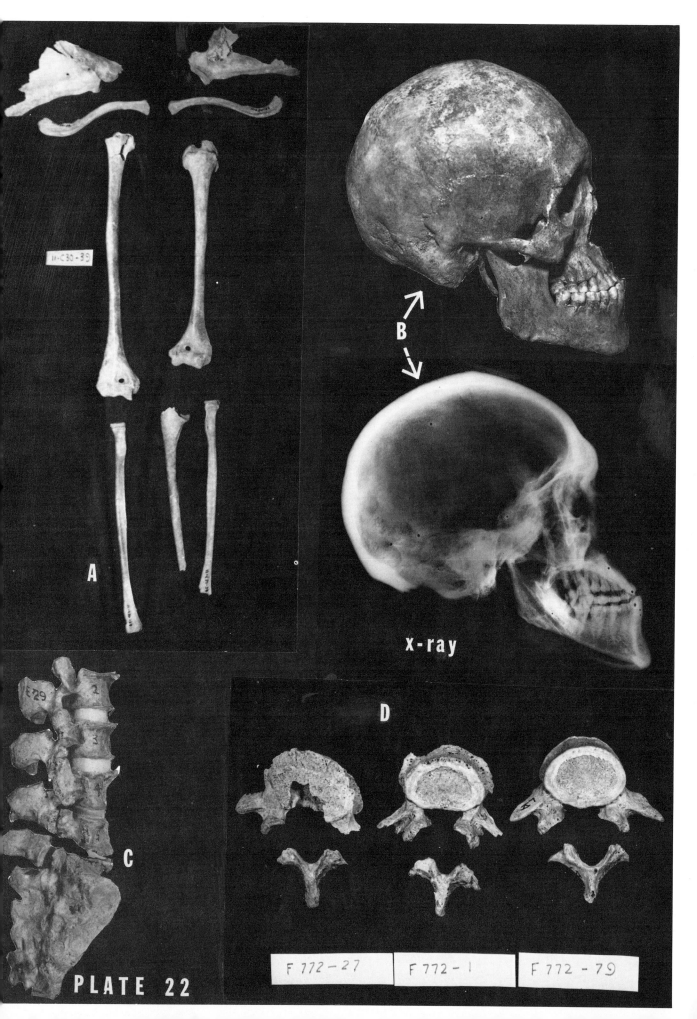

x-ray

PLATE 22

F 772-27   F 772-1   F 772-79

PLATE 23

ANOMALIES

A. The right tibia and fibula were shorter than the left, probably due to a traumatic injury to the nerve during the growing period with a paralysis of the right lower leg involving the foot. There is a facet (arrow) on the anterior lateral surface of the tibia. The heel would have been inverted. This location is where one finds a "squatting facet." In this case, however, the facet resulted because of the foot deformity. Burial No. 287, Male, age 30 (See Plate 5,H). Dickson Mound (F34), Fulton Co., Ill. Mississippian Culture.

B. Spina bifida involving all sacral segments. The fifth lumbar vertebra is normal. Burial No. 473, Male, age 46. Dickson Mound (F34), Fulton Co., Ill. Mississippian Culture.

C. Perforated olecranon fossa. This is a rather common anomaly and occurs much more frequently in females. Burial No. 25, Female, age 29. Morse Site (F772), Fulton Co., Ill. Red Ocher Culture (Late Archaic).

D. Skull from Arkansas showing binding deformation. Mississippian Culture.

E. Cradleboard deformation. Crable Site, Fulton Co., Ill. Mississippian Culture.

F. Posterior view of skull showing severe pitting in occipital bone. Similar pitting in the orbits is called cribia orbitalia. Probably from Crable Site, Fulton Co., Ill. Dickson Mounds Collection.

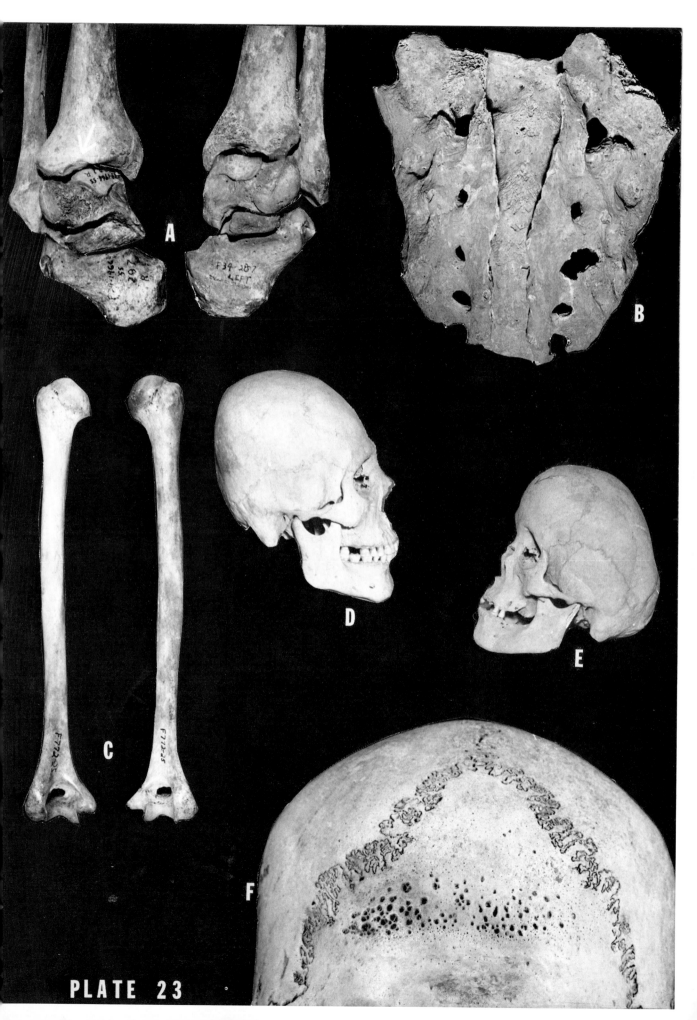

PLATE 23

PLATE 24

ANOMALIES

A.   Microcephalic. Male, age 14. Riviere aux Vase Site, Macomb Co., Mich. Late Woodland Culture. *Photograph, courtesy Museum of Anthropology, University of Michigan.*

B.   Hydrocephalic. The exact age is questionable. From tooth eruption, the age appears to be about 6. From length of the long bones, the age is determined to be 3 years and 4 months (Maresh 1955). Emmons Farm, Fulton Co., Ill. Red Ocher Culture (Late Archaic).

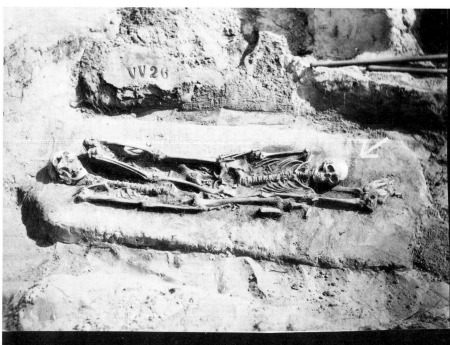

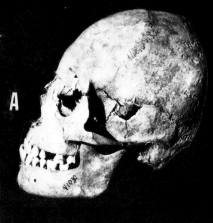

A

inch

Microcephalic

L : 141
H : 108
B : 124

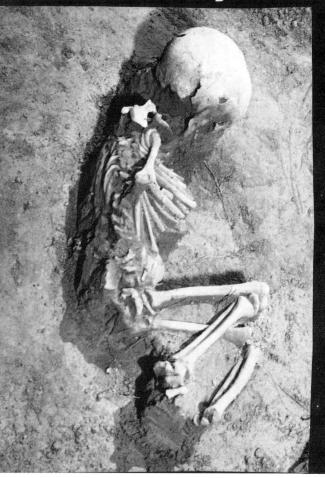

B

Hydrocephalic

L : 172
H : 148
B : 148

Adult Male Indian
Length : 180 mm
Height : 150 mm
Breadth : 136 mm

PLATE 24

PLATE 25

DENTAL PATHOLOGY

A. Example of tooth filing of left upper and lower central permanent incisors. The filing was done in a matching diamond-shaped cut of equal depth on both teeth. Dick's Mound, Adams Co., Ill. Late Woodland Culture. Collection of Dr. James Reed, Quincy, Illinois.

B. Multiple notches filed on incisor teeth as seen in this figure are somewhat rare in Mississippian Culture and more common in Mexico. Cahokia Site, Ill. Mississippian Culture. (Holder and Stewart 1958). *Photograph, courtesy Joe Berta.*

C. Bilateral occurrence of two supernumerary premolars reduced in form and size. The two on the left were lost postmortem. The marked wear on the lower incisor teeth indicates some unusual use other than simple biting or chewing. Many primitive populations are known to use their incisor teeth as tools. Berry Site, Fulton Co., Ill. Mississippian Culture. Dickson Mounds Collection.

D. A pearl of enamel sometimes forms as terminal activity of the enamel producing cells in a tooth's development. The absence of the upper right second molar allows the pearl to be seen clearly in the anterior surface of the upper third molar. Such structures are found principally in the molar teeth, and on some occasions the cells involved continue up a short distance on the tooth's surface leaving a fine line or trail of enamel. Found on surface, Emmons Village Site, Fulton Co., Ill. Mississippian Culture.

E. Excessive function and irritants such as heavy calculary deposits around the gum margins of the teeth sometimes stimulate the adjacent bone to activity, producing a ledge or lipping of new bone as seen on the buccal surface of the distal root of the lower right second molar. Note the peculiar wear pattern on the first and second molars. The first molar wear is far advanced over that of the second due to its strategic functional position plus the fact that it was in use for six years before the second molar erupted and became functional. Weaver Site, Fulton Co., Ill. Hopewell Culture. Dickson Mounds Collection.

F. The first permanent molar tooth is most often the target and victim of heavy usage where abrasive foods are used. This tooth functions as the principal masticating unit for many years while the deciduous (primary) teeth are being lost and before the replacements become functional. A pit on the buccal surface of lower molars is commonplace among Indians. This is seen on the third molar. On the second molar a distal deviation of the buccal groove in its gingeval third is to be noted. Crable Site, Fulton Co., Ill. Mississippian Culture. Dickson Mounds Collection (K1405).

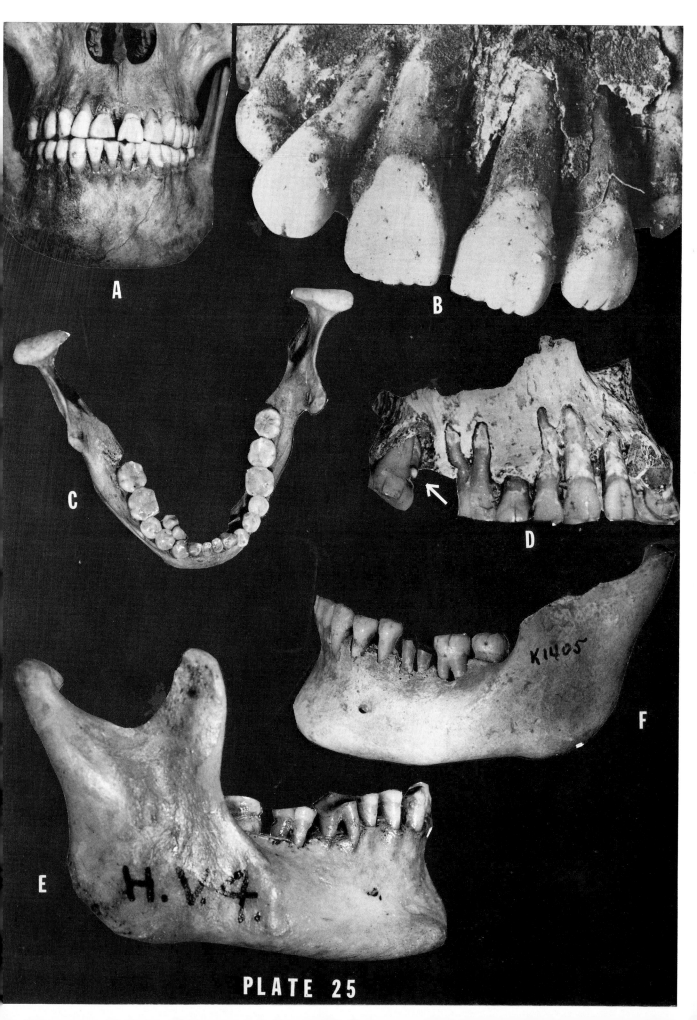

PLATE 25

PLATE 26

DENTAL PATHOLOGY

A. This individual at thirteen years of age had beautiful alignment and presentation of permanent teeth due in part to a good balance of bone support and tooth size. This is contrasted sharply by the dentition illustrated in H, where the teeth were too large for the amount of supporting bone available in the jaws. Female, age 13. Crable Site, Fulton Co., Ill. Mississippian Culture. Dickson Mounds Collection (635).

B. Teeth sometimes develop in unusual positions and erupt outside their normal areas of function. In this instance the upper permanent right central incisor was reversed in its developmental position and took a direction toward the floor of the nose. Burial No. 5, Male, age 20. Dickson Mound (F34), Fulton Co., Ill. Mississippian Culture.

C. Another example of malposition of a tooth in the development phase. The lower third molar erupted toward the inferior border of the mandible. The specimen is viewed from the lingual with the first permanent molar in its proper alveolar position. Right half of mandible. Dickson Mounds Collection.

D. X-ray view of the portion of right mandible in C. The two teeth are fully a quarter inch apart, a second molar might have been present but, if so, healing of the bone would indicate that it had been lost or removed many years antemortem.

E. The sharp spinous ridge on the alveolar processes of the upper and lower jaws indicate that the teeth were lost many years prior to the death of this individual (Note comments on G). Female, age 65. Crable Site, Fulton Co., Ill. Mississippian Culture. Dickson Mounds Collection (K6941).

F. This individual experienced an acute alveolar abscess in the upper right canine area resulting in swelling and pain on the right side of the face and in the right palate. The condition of the bone edges of the resulting sinus in the palate indicates that the condition resolved and healed itself. The offending tooth was not lost in the episode but remained through the individual's entire life and was lost postmortem. Other teeth were lost antemortem with good healing of the sockets. Burial No. 23, Male, age 45. Dickson Mound (F34), Fulton Co., Ill. Mississippian Culture.

G. X-ray of skull illustrated in E. A piece of root is seen in the lower canine region.

H. Severe crowding of upper and lower teeth due to the excessive amount of tooth material for the limited amount of bone available to support or carry the teeth. On the left upper side there is also a supernumerary lateral incisor tooth. All the incisor teeth show ridges on the lingual surfaces. This condition is referred to as shovel-shaped. In this individual the upper central incisors had ridges on the lateral aspects of the labial surface as well. This ridging of two surfaces on a tooth makes it double shovel-shaped. Female, age 17. Crable Site, Fulton Co., Ill. Mississippian Culture.

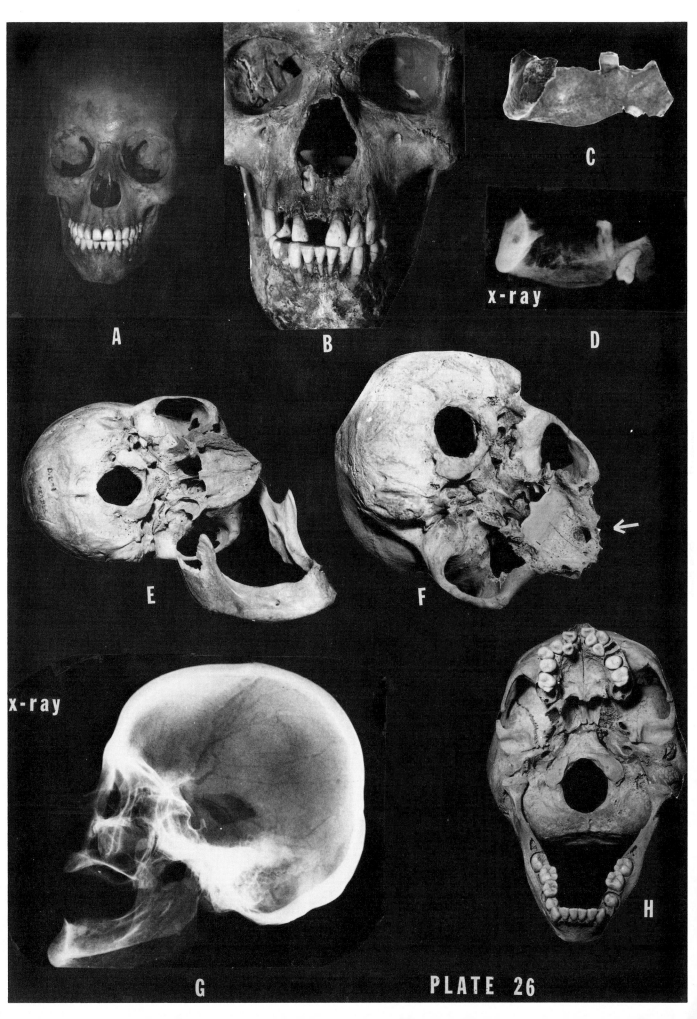

A

B

C

x-ray

D

E

F

x-ray

G

H

PLATE 26

PLATE 27

DENTAL PATHOLOGY

A. Rather marked exostosis is seen on the buccal aspect of the alveolar ridge of the maxilla. This was a response of the bone to the inflammatory condition which existed in association with the alveolar abscess which had existed around the third molar and the heavy calculous deposits (now removed) which had impinged upon the gingeval tissues. Dickson Mound (F34), Fulton Co., Ill. Mississippian Culture.

B. An unusual cleft of the left maxilla. There is evidence of minimal bone regeneration, indicating that the condition existed prior to death. Indian Mound Park, Adams Co., Ill. Late Woodland Culture. Collection of Dr. James Reed, Quincy, Illinois.

C. Early loss of the mandibular posterior teeth is contrasted with more recent loss (antemortem) of the upper posterior teeth in this individual. In the absence of posterior teeth the owner of this dentition performed all functions of mastication on the incisor teeth. Crable Site, Fulton Co., Ill. Mississippian Culture. Dickson Mounds Collection.

D. Effects of wear are seen on this jaw. The horseshoe appearance of dentin in the worn incisor shows the structural aspect of the sturdy shovel-shaped teeth. The right lateral incisor in this individual lacked the shovel shape but had the rounded character or what is called the barrel shape, the counterpart of the peg shape found in other population groups. Note caries of second premolar and second molar on the left. Crable Site, Fulton Co., Ill. Mississippian Culture. Dickson Mounds Collection.

E. This right half of the maxilla illustrates the ridging common to Indian dentitions. The accentuation gives the central and lateral incisors the appearance of shovels, hence, the name, shovel-shaped incisors. The irregularities of bone in the palate are not pathologic, but are adaptations about the blood vessels and tissues of the palate. Crable Site, Fulton Co., Ill. Mississippian Culture. Dickson Mounds Collection.

F. Unusual attrition of the mesial surface of the first and second upper permanent molars is seen without matching attrition facets on the associated contacting surfaces. The maxillary canine is misplaced, being posterior to the first premolar rather than anterior. This caused the second premolar to be crowded out of its normal position. Peter's Mound, Fulton Co., Ill. Late Woodland Culture. Dickson Mounds Collection.

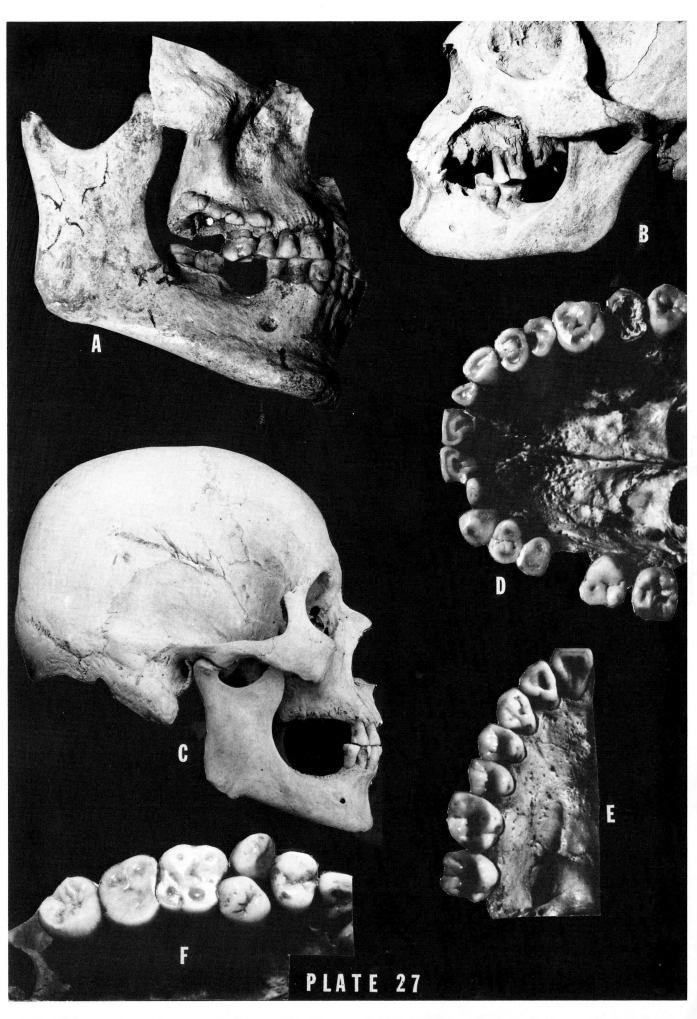

PLATE 27

PLATE 28

PREHISTORIC HUNCHBACK ART FORMS IN AMERICA

UPPER LEFT AND LOWER CENTER: Examples of the many severe spinal deformities among the residents of Lincoln State School, illustrating that kyphosis is not synonymous with spinal tuberculosis. (Interpretation of the roentgenograms made by Dr. Edward Wood, consulting radiologist at Lincoln State School.)

A. Wedging of vertebral bodies and marginal spurring.

B. Compression deformity of thoracic vertebrae with no actual bone lesion.

C. Fusion of several vertebral bodies suggesting a lack of segmentation.

D. No significant bone changes.

LOWER LEFT: Pictograph of hunchbacked flute players, Arizona. (B.A.E. Bull. 65, Smithsonian Institution)

UPPER RIGHT: Hunchbacked water bottles from Memphis area.

A & B. Side and front view of figure representing an old "crone" (toothless old woman). Found with Burial No. 70, Banks Site, Crittenden Co., Ark. Obtained by Gregory Perino for the Gilcrease Foundation.

C. Vessel height, 7½ in. From Mississippi Co., Mo. Found by Gray LaDassor, St. Louis, Mo. Gilcrease Foundation Collection.

D. Vessel height, 6½ in. Note smooth curve of the hunch. Bradley Site, Crittenden Co., Ark. Found by T. W. Gitchell, West Memphis, Ark. Dan Morse Collection.

E. Male with bulging chest. Note the five spinous processes. Found with Burial No. 244 along with three other vessels. Banks Site, Crittenden Co., Ark. Obtained by Gregory Perino. Gilcrease Foundation Collection.

F. Vessel height, 6 in. Mississippi Co., Mo. Found by Gray LaDassor, St. Louis, Mo. Gilcrease Foundation Collection.

G. Knots on the back may represent a pack. Figure is seated on a "throne." Height, 7¾ in. New Madrid Co., Mo. Gilcrease Foundation Collection.

H. Silver figure of a man on a llama. Height, 4½ in. From Cuzco, Peru, Incan Culture (USNM Cat. No. 210366) *Photograph, courtesy Smithsonian Institution.*

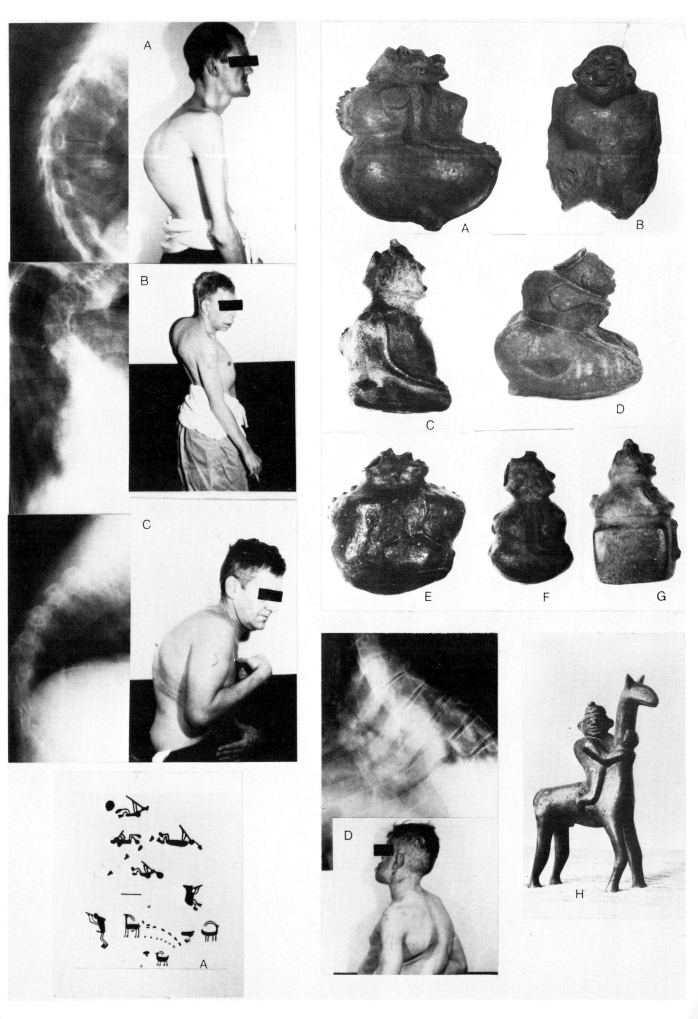

PLATE 29

PREHISTORIC AMERICAN SPINAL DISEASE

A. Case 2. Found by Clarence B. Moore in 1913 in a mound at Sorrel Bayou, Iberville Parish, Louisiana. (USNM Cat. No. 277730) *Photograph, courtesy of Division of Physical Anthropology, U. S. National Museum.*

B. Case 6. Excavated in 1938 in a cemetery in Livingston County, New York, by William Ritchie and Charles Wray. (Rochester Museum Cat. No. AP 526). *Photograph, courtesy of Rochester Museum of Arts and Sciences and Dr. William A. Ritchie.*

C. Case 9. Found by Lloyd Gordon O'Bannon in Montgomery Co., Tennessee. (USNM Cat. No. 381212). *Photograph, courtesy of Division of Physical Anthropology, U.S. National Museum.*

D. Case 15. Found by Rod Hiles near Frederick, Illinois. Dickson Mounds Collection.

E. Case 13. Discovered by Glen McGirr in the early 1930's at Crable Site, Fulton County, Illinois.

F. Case 14. Excavated by Merrill Emmons and Dan F. Morse at the Emmons Cemetery, Fulton County, Illinois.

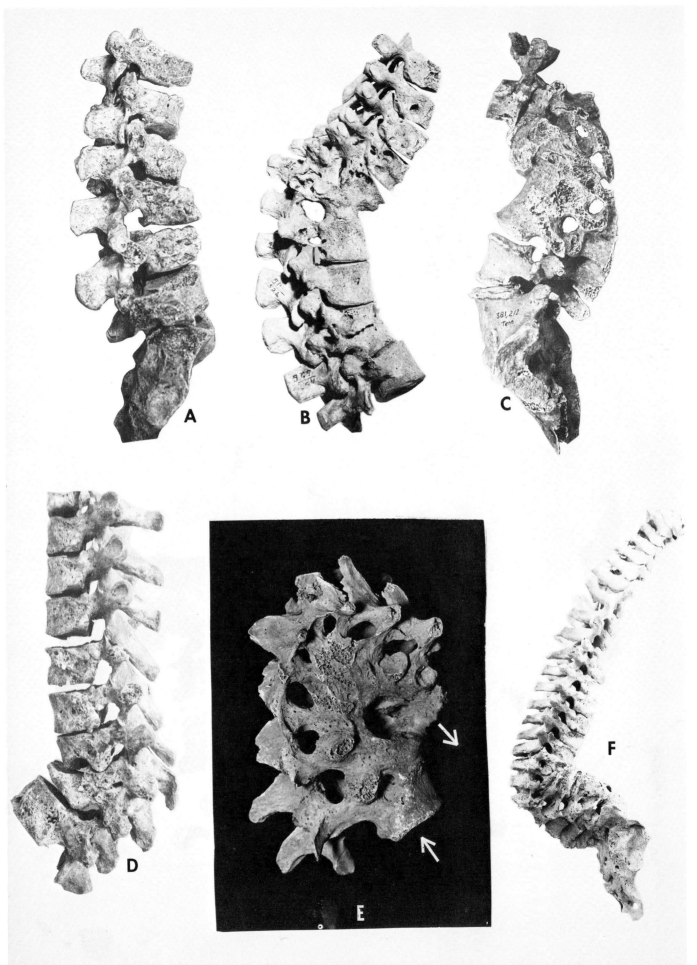

PLATE 29

PLATE 30

TREPONEMA INFECTION

A. Case 1. Osteitis involving the frontal bone and extensive destruction of the skeletal portion of the mid-face (gangosa). Rose Mounds,
Schuyler Co., Ill. Mississippian Culture.

B. Case 1. Anterior surface of the left tibia. Pronounced periostitis
and osteomyelitis of the kind seen in yaws and syphilis.

C. Case 2. Microscopic sections of an involved rib. See text for description. Thompson Site, Fulton Co., Ill. Early Mississippian Culture.

D. Case 2. Subperiosteal thickening and erosion of the anterior surface
of the frontal bone.

E. Case 2. Slight bone destruction with a predominant bony proliferation forming multiple nodules. This lesion is different in character
from the disease process found in other bones. The nodules are
located on the sacrum and the greater trochanter of the right femur
and involve points of subcutaneous bony prominence which are common sites of decubitus ulceration. The pathology was probably the
result of pressure and infection (bedsore).

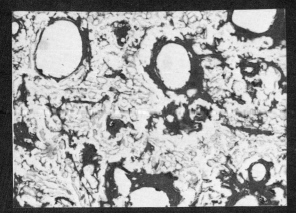

x 100

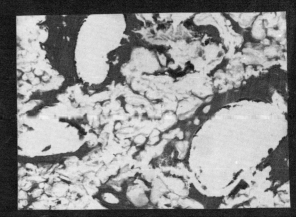

x 200

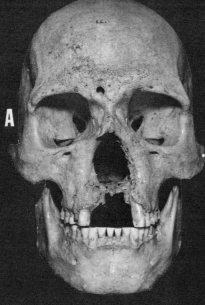

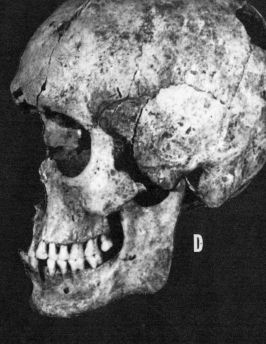

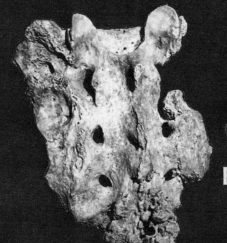

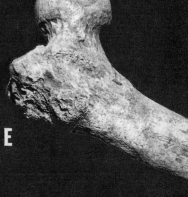

PLATE 30

PLATE 31

TREPONEMA INFECTION

A-E: Case 1. Rose Mound, Schuyler Co., Ill. Mississippian Culture.

A & B: Skull and maxilla show a partial destruction of the palate and the anterior alveolar area.

C & D: Severe osteitis of the distal end of the left humerus, proximal end of the right ulna, and the outer half of the superior surface of the left clavicle.

W-Z: Case 2. Thompson Site, Fulton Co., Ill. Mississippian Culture.

W.   Osteitis of the frontal bone.

X & Z.   Osteomyelitis with sinus formation of the distal end of the left femur and the upper end of the shaft of the right ulna.

Y.   The same disease process involves the distal portion of the right humerus with sinus formation and corcical erosion. The entire bone seems shortened. There appears to have been an old fracture at its distal third. This fracture may have been pathological or could be unrelated to the main disease.

Art work by Alan Harn

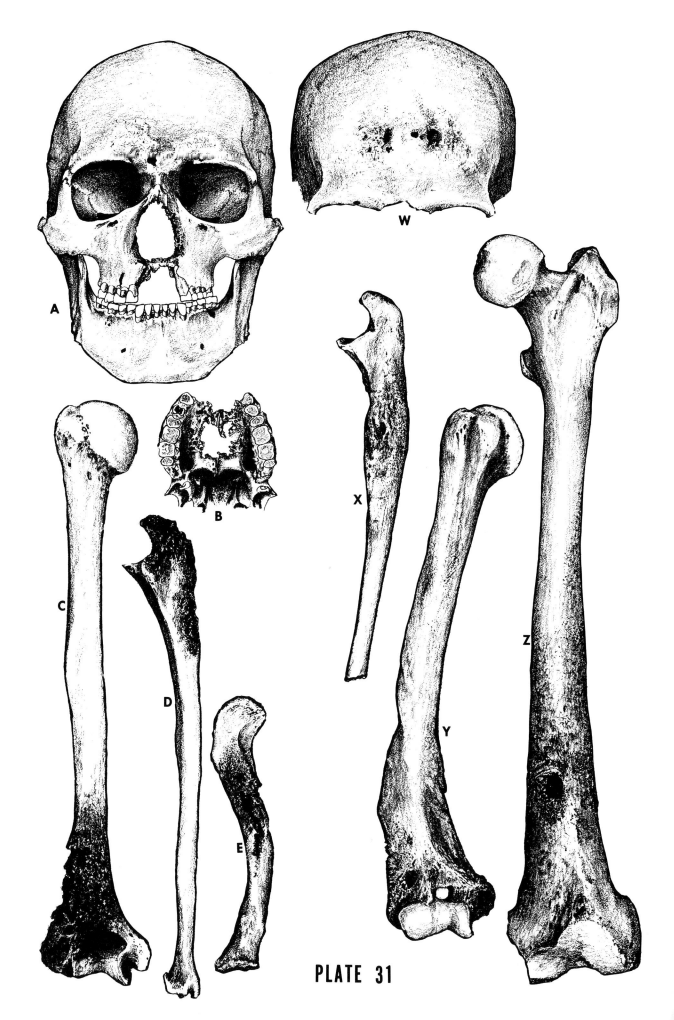

PLATE 31

PLATE 32

KIDNEY STONE AND MULTIPLE MYELOMA

A. Burial No. 18 was in a flexed position; near the arms was a full-term fetus, suggesting that childbirth may have been the cause of death. Associated grave goods were a blue-white granite boatstone and an unfinished large galena bead, shown just above the right iliac crest in the photograph. Female, age 20. Morse Site (F707), Fulton Co., Ill. Red Ocher Culture (Late Archaic). Excavated by Dr. Georg K. Neumann, Indiana University.

B. A kidney or bladder stone was found among the removed bones after Burial No. 18 was taken to the laboratory for study. This is not seen in Photograph A. The stone was bean-shaped and measured 10 by 8 by 5 mm.

C. The stone was examined by Dr. Carl Beck, Department of Geology, Indiana University. X-ray defraction analysis was performed (lower graph C) and the stone was determined to be apatite, $Ca_{10}(PO_4)_6(OH)_2$. The upper graph in C represents the results of an x-ray defraction analysis of a similar stone found with a burial on the Bowen Site (Ft. Ancient Culture), Marion County, Indiana.

D. and F. are x-rays, and E. is a photograph of a case of multiple myeloma found in California. The following information was graciously supplied by Albert B. Elsasser, Assistant Research Anthropologist of the University of California, Berkeley: "The specimen is located in the R. H. Lowie Museum of Anthropology (Cat. No. 12-4356). The burial was excavated by Ronald L. Olson in 1928. The occupation site is known simply as Site 100, Santa Cruz Island, and the depth of the deposit in which the material was found is noted as 42 inches. The estimated date of the occupation is somewhere between A.D. 300 to A.D. 1450 (Late Horizon). The results of the excavation are described briefly in Olson, 1930." *Photographs, courtesy of the Lowie Museum, Department of Anthropology, University of California, Berkeley.*

A case of multiple myeloma similar to the one from California, from the Kane Site (Mississippian Culture), Madison County, Illinois, is described in detail by Brooks and Melbye, 1967.

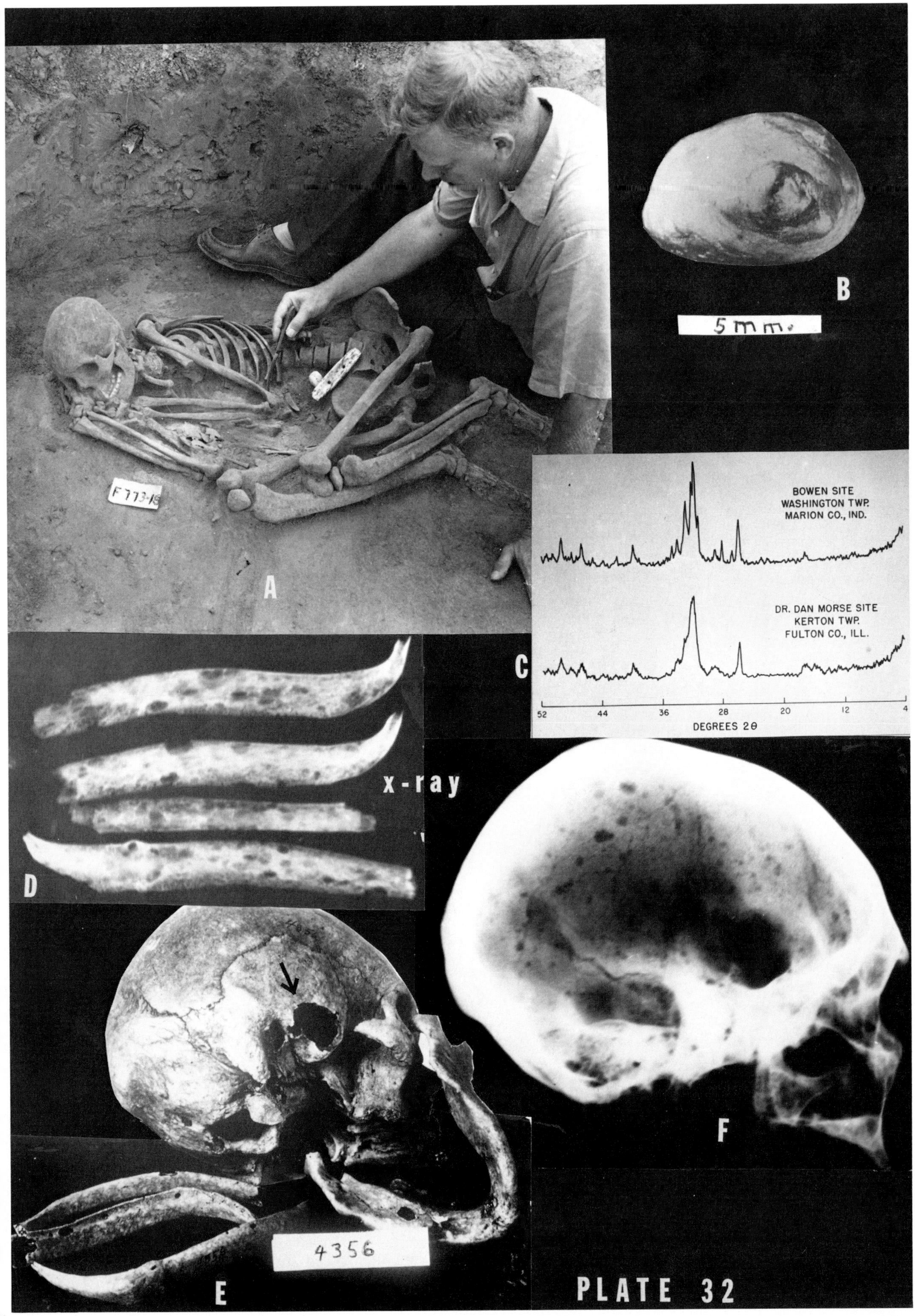
A
B
5 mm.
C
BOWEN SITE
WASHINGTON TWP.
MARION CO., IND.
DR. DAN MORSE SITE
KERTON TWP.
FULTON CO., ILL.
52 44 36 28 20 12 4
DEGREES 2θ
x-ray
D
E
4356
F

PLATE 32

PLATE 33

PATHOLOGY OF THE ROBINSON SITE SKELETONS
(Sm4, Smith Co., Tenn.)

A. Vault thickening and pitting of the surface of the anterior portion of the frontal and upper part of both parietal bones. This bone reaction was probably due to an adjacent soft tissue infection which may have originated from a large opening (arrow) in the frontal sinus and spread over the anterior portion of the scalp. Burial No. 43, Male, age 40.

B. There is a bilateral follicular cyst-like indentation on the interior posterior surface of each ramus of the mandible (Harvey and Noble, 1968). The defect on the left is the larger (arrow). Photographs and x-rays of this specimen were sent to Dr. Warren Harvey of the Dental School of the University of Glasgow. Dr. Harvey had been making a special study of mandibular defects and reports in a personal letter to the author that the anomaly in Burial No. 52 is exactly like the five cases he has seen in an examination of 973 dry mandibles. [Four out of 186 lower jaws from India; one of 177 (1696-1852) English; none from 35 of different races, and none from 575 Stone Age to Medieval British mandibles.] Moss and Levey 1966, reviewed the literature on this subject and reported three cases of mandibular cysts following trauma. It would seem that there is a great deal of confusion concerning these cysts of the lower jaw and there is need for additional clarification in regard to their classification, pathology and etiology. Burial No. 52, Female, age 50.

C. Osteoarthritis of the interphalangeal joint of the great toe of the left foot. Burial No. 11, Female, age 30.

D. There is a hole into each antrum to admit the root of the second molar. The wall of the right maxillary sinus is thickened because of a chronic sinusitis. Burial No. 55, Female, age 45.

E. Impacted third right upper molar. The partially erupted right canine is deflected laterally. Burial No. 9, Female, age 30.

F. Pitting erosion and swelling of an area of bone in the left parietal along the course of the middle meningeal artery. These changes are visible both on the internal and external surfaces. Burial No. 31, Female, age 50+.

G. An inflammatory reaction as evidenced by subperiosteal new bone formation involving the left side of the mandible, the maxilla and extending backward to the region of the external auditory meatus. Burial No. 58, Female, age 22.

H. Healed fracture of proximal end of the right femur and fracture (healed) of the right tibia at the junction of the upper and middle thirds. A bony bridge connects the tibia and fibula. Burial No. 5, Female, age 29.

Examination of the Robinson Site skeletons was through the courtesy of Dr. Alfred K. Guthe, Head of the Department of Anthropology, University of Tennessee.

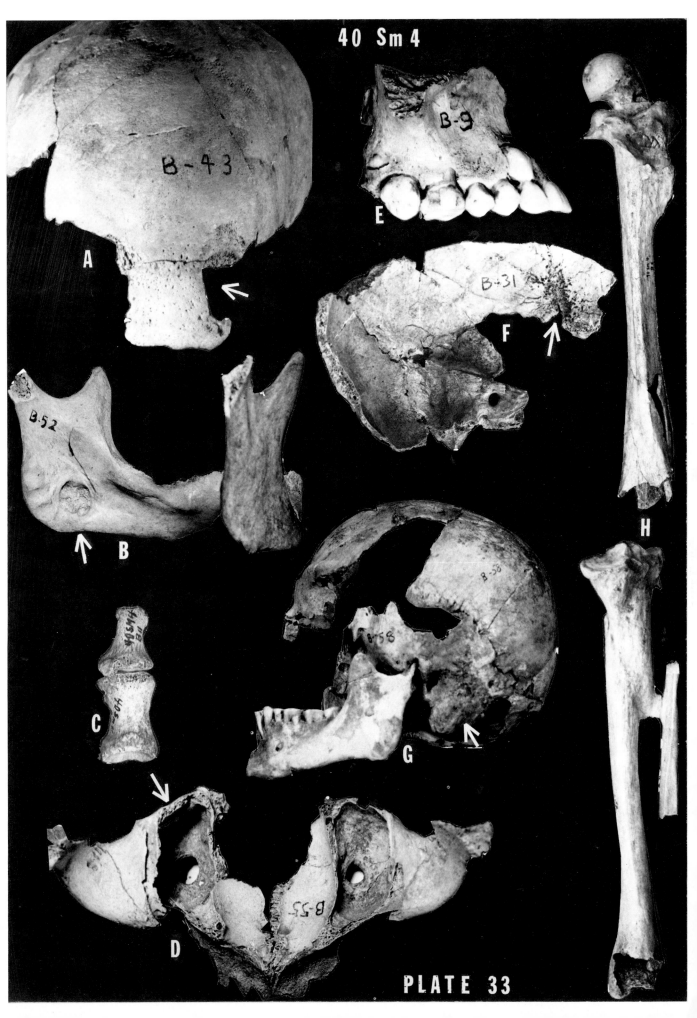

40 Sm 4

PLATE 33

PLATE 34

X-RAYS OF THE ROBINSON SITE PATHOLOGY

(Sm4, Smith Co., Tenn.)

A. The lower half of the right humerus is enlarged and flattened with distortion of the articular surface. The same sclerotic inflammatory changes are seen in the right ulna and to a lesser degree in the right radius. Burial No. 4, Male, age 26.

B. X-rays of Burial No. 5. See Plate 33,H.

C. X-rays of mandibles and maxillae of Burial Nos. 9, 25, and 55.
Burial No. 25 is a 13-year-old adolescent. Both lower wisdom teeth are unerupted and impacted.
Burial No. 9 has impacted molar and crowded canine.
Burial No. 55 demonstrates chronic sinusitis on the right maxilla.

D. X-rays of Burial Nos. 31, 11, and 52.
Burial No. 31, interior left parietal. See Plate 33,F.
Burial No. 11, arthritic great toe.
Burial No. 52, cyst, right mandibular ramus.

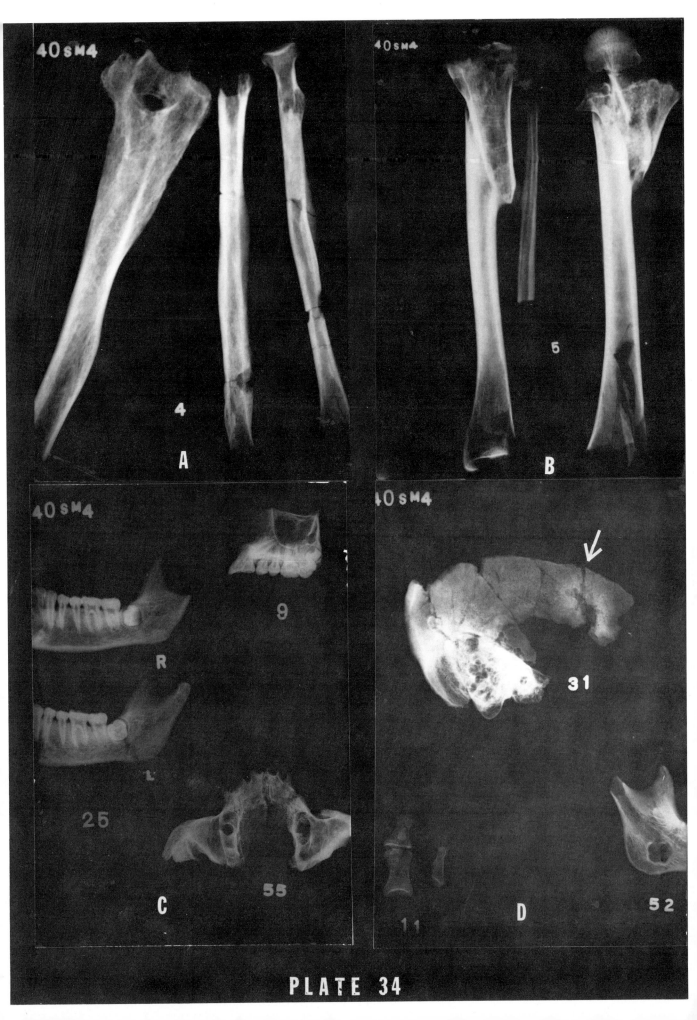

PLATE 34

PLATE 35

DICKSON MOUND

A portion of the area of Dickson Mound showing burials *in situ*. These are permanently on exhibit in one wing of the new (1970) museum at Dickson Mounds. Insert, upper right, the late Don F. Dickson.

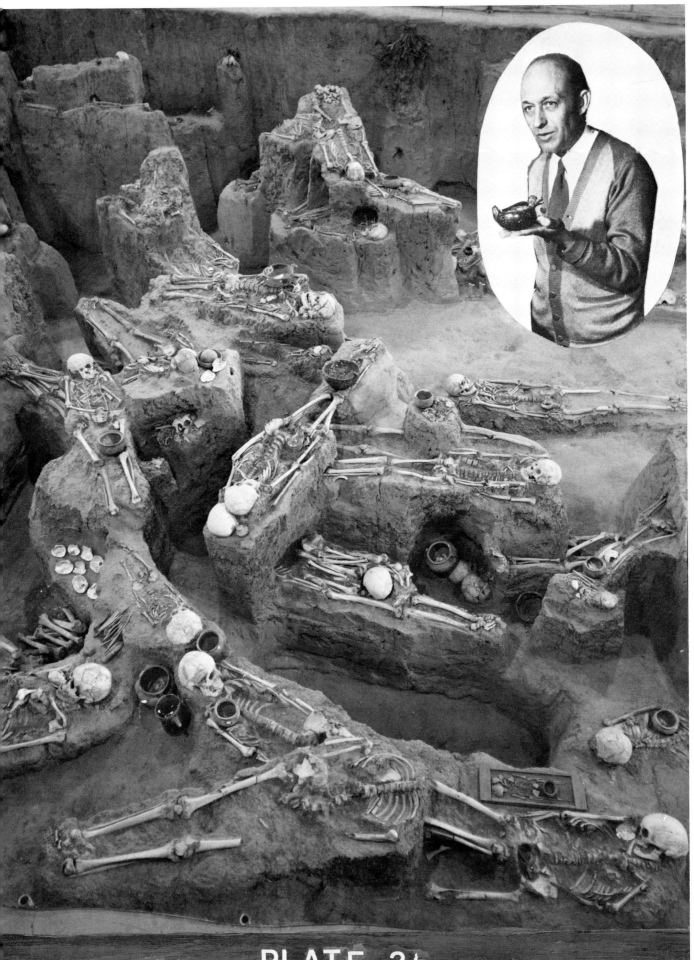

PLATE 35

PLATE 36

CRABLE SITE, FULTON COUNTY, ILLINOIS

UPPER: These two photographs, taken during the 1964 excavation by the Department of Anthropology, Indiana University, demonstrate the construction history of the "Temple" mound. The configuration of the post molds in the photo on the right suggests that a circular structure, possibly forty-seven feet in diameter, existed when the mound was first started. In the left photograph Dr. Georg Neumann, field director of the project, points to one of the five floors (seen in the profile) made by the Indians during the time the mound was in use. The mottled area below Dr. Neumann's hand is evidence of "loading" (depositing dirt by the basket-load).

LOWER: Some typical Mississippian artifacts from the Crable Site. The length of the small arrow points on the right would average about one inch.

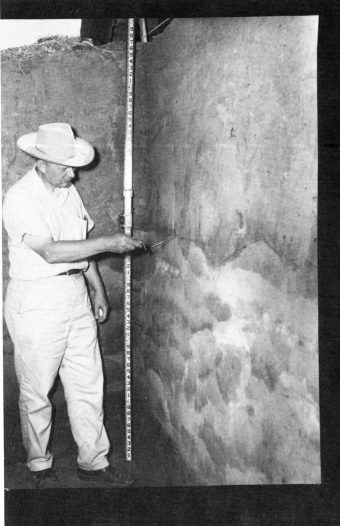

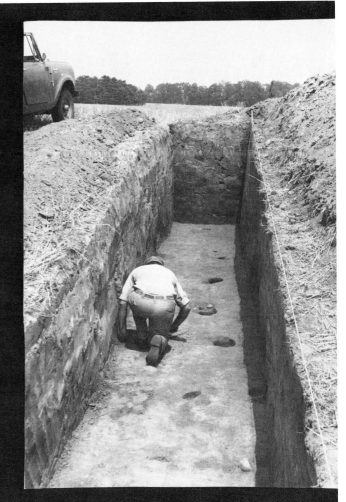

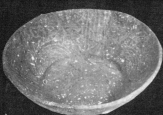

plate

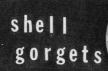

**shell
gorgets**

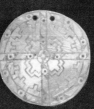

bowl

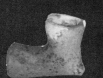

pipe

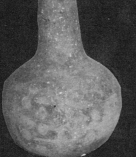

bottle

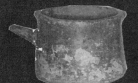

beaker

PLATE 36

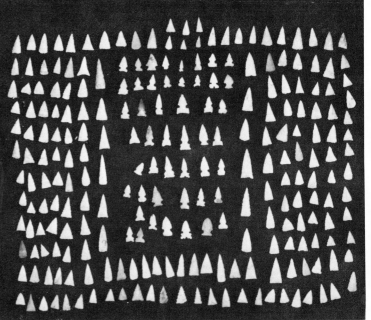

PLATE 37

TOMOGRAPHY

A. Photograph of a skull (female age 42) showing extensive osteitis and periostitis over almost all of the frontal bone. Hampson Museum specimen #843, Wilson, Arkansas. Late Mississippi culture-circa A. D. 1400–1700. (See Dan Morse 1973.)

B. Posterior (posterior of skull is closest to the film) view of skull.

C. Lateral x-ray showing no particular abnormality. The frontal bone seems to be within the limits of normal.

D. Tomograms taken at levels 7, 7½ and 8 cm. These show a diseased area of the frontal bone extending into the parietal. There is a thickening of the cranial wall, erosion of both the inner and outer tables and penetration (arrow). These tomograms are valuable because they show much more than the posterior and lateral x-rays and even more than visual examination of the bone specimen itself.

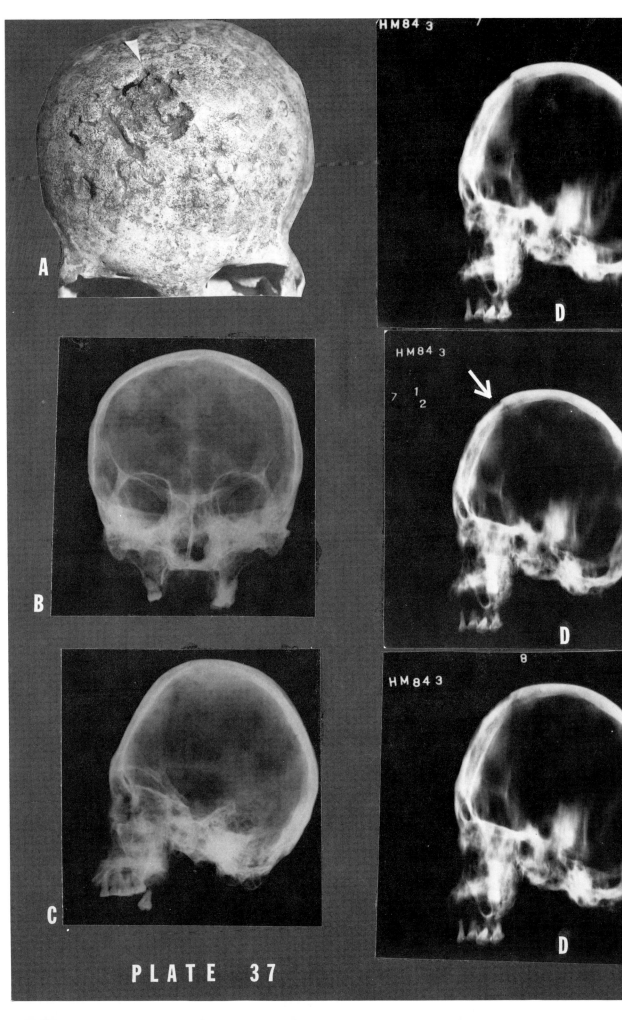

PLATE 37

mls 47